Atlas of
INFECTIOUS DISEASES

Volume IX

URINARY TRACT INFECTIONS AND INFECTIONS OF THE FEMALE PELVIS

Atlas of
INFECTIOUS DISEASES

Volume IX

URINARY TRACT INFECTIONS AND INFECTIONS OF THE FEMALE PELVIS

Editor-in-Chief

Gerald L. Mandell, MD

Professor of Medicine
Owen R. Cheatham Professor of the Sciences
Chief, Division of Infectious Diseases
University of Virginia Health Sciences Center
Charlottesville, Virginia

Editor

Jack D. Sobel, MD

Professor of Medicine
Wayne State University School of Medicine
Chief of Infectious Diseases
Harper Hospital
Detroit, Michigan

With 15 contributors

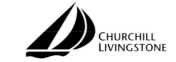

CHURCHILL
LIVINGSTONE

DEVELOPED BY CURRENT MEDICINE, INC.
PHILADELPHIA

CURRENT MEDICINE
400 MARKET STREET, SUITE 700
PHILADELPHIA, PA 19106

Library of Congress Cataloging-in-Publication Data

Urinary tract infections and infections of the female pelvis / editor-in-chief, Gerald L. Mandell; editor Jack D. Sobel.
     p. cm.–(Atlas of infectious diseases ; v. 9)
   Includes bibliographical references and index.
   ISBN 0-443-07770-3 (hardcover)
   1. Urinary tract infections. 2. Pelvis—Infections.
3. Women—Diseases. I. Mandell, Gerald L. II. Sobel, Jack D. III. Series.
   [DNLM: 1. Urinary Tract Infections—atlases. 2. Genital Diseases, Female—atlases.
WJ 17 U76 1997]
RG484.U74 1997
616.6—dc20
DNLM/DLC
for Library of Congress
       96-24706
       CIP

Development Editors:	Lee Tevebaugh and Michael Bokulich
Editorial Assistant:	Elena Coler
Art Director:	Paul Fennessy
Design and Layout:	Patrick Ward, Lisa Weischedel, and Christine M. Keller
Illustration Director:	Ann Saydlowski
Illustrators:	Elizabeth Carrozza, Beth Starkey, Gary Welch, and Wieslawa Langenfeld
Production:	David Myers and Lori Holland
Managing Editor:	Lori J. Bainbridge
Indexer:	Ann Cassar

Printed in Hong Kong by Paramount Printing Group Limited.

10 9 8 7 6 5 4 3 2 1

PREFACE

The diagnosis and management of patients with infectious diseases are based in large part on visual clues. Skin and mucous membrane lesions, eye findings, imaging studies, Gram stains, culture plates, insect vectors, preparations of blood, urine, pus, cerebrospinal fluid, and biopsy specimens are studied to establish the proper diagnosis and to choose the most effective therapy. The *Atlas of Infectious Diseases* is a modern, complete collection of these images. Current Medicine, with its capability of superb color reproduction and its state-of-the-art computer imaging facilities, is the ideal publisher for the atlas. Infectious diseases physicians, scientists, microbiologists, and pathologists frequently teach other health-care professionals, and this comprehensive atlas with available slides is an effective teaching tool.

Dr. Jack Sobel is an infectious diseases authority with special knowledge and experience in clinical and research aspects of urinary tract infections and gynecologic infections. He has assembled a group of experts who have prepared instructive and informative chapters. The images are truly outstanding, and this volume will be very useful for clinicians, educators, and researchers.

Gerald L. Mandell, MD
Charlottesville, Virginia

CONTRIBUTORS

Michel G. Bergeron, MD, FRCPC
Professor and Chairman
Department of Microbiology
Laval University Faculty of Medicine
Microbiologist
Centre Hospitalier de L'Université Laval
Québec City, Québec
Canada

Claude Delage, MD, FRCPC
Professor of Pathology
Laval University Faculty of Medicine
Pathologist
L'Hôtel-Dieu de Québec Hospital
Québec City, Québec
Canada

Harry A. Gallis, MD
Clinical Professor of Medicine
Department of Internal Medicine
University of North Carolina School of Medicine
Chapel Hill, North Carolina
Vice President, Regional Medical Education
Carolinas Healthcare System
Charlotte, North Carolina

Dominique Giroux, MD, FRCP
Lecturer
Department of Radiology
Laval University Faculty of Medicine
Radiologist
L'Hôtel-Dieu de Québec Hospital
Québec City, Québec
Canada

Elaine T. Kaye, MD
Clinical Instructor
Department of Dermatology
Harvard Medical School
Assistant in Medicine
Children's Hospital Medical Center
Boston, Massachusetts

Edward D. Kim, MD
Assistant Professor
Scott Department of Urology
Baylor College of Medicine
Houston, Texas

J. Curtis Nickel, MD, FRCSC
Professor of Urology
Queen's University
Kingston General Hospital
Kingston, Ontario
Canada

Lindsay E. Nicolle, MD, FRCPC
H.E. Seller Professor and Chair
Department of Internal Medicine
University of Manitoba
Health Sciences Centre
St. Boniface General Hospital
Winnipeg, Manitoba
Canada

Paul Nyirjesy, MD
Assistant Professor
Departments of Obstetrics, Gynecology, & Reproductive
  Sciences and Medicine
Temple University School of Medicine
Philadelphia, Pennsylvania

Anthony J. Schaeffer, MD
Herman L. Kretschmer Professor and Chairman
Department of Urology
Northwestern University Medical School
Northwestern Medical Faculty Foundation, Inc.
Chicago, Illinois

Jack D. Sobel, MD
Professor of Medicine
Wayne State University School of Medicine
Chief of Infectious Diseases
Harper Hospital
Detroit, Michigan

David E. Soper, MD
Professor
Departments of Obstetrics & Gynecology and Medicine
Division of Infectious Diseases
Medical University of South Carolina
Charleston, South Carolina

Richard L. Sweet, MD
Professor and Chair
Department of Obstetrics, Gynecology, and
  Reproductive Sciences
University of Pittsburgh School of Medicine/Magee-
  Women's Hospital
Pittsburgh, Pennsylvania

Harold C. Wiesenfeld, MD, CM
Assistant Professor
Department of Obstetrics, Gynecology, and
  Reproductive Sciences
University of Pittsburgh School of Medicine/Magee-
  Women's Hospital
Co-Director
Sexually Transmitted Diseases Program
Allegheny County Health Department
Pittsburgh, Pennsylvania

Edward S. Wong, MD
Associate Professor of Medicine
Medical College of Virginia
Chief, Infectious Diseases Section
McGuire Veterans Affairs Hospital
Richmond, Virginia

CONTENTS

CHAPTER 1

Cystitis

Edward S. Wong

EPIDEMIOLOGY AND PATHOGENESIS

Epidemiology of bacterial cystitis

20%–30% of women experience an episode of cystitis during
  their lifetime
~20% of women experience recurrent infections
Recurrent infections are often clustered: two thirds occur within
  6 months
Annually, in the United States, bacterial cystitis accounts for:
  7 million visits to physicians' offices
  1% of clinic visits
  $1 billion in outpatient care costs

FIGURE 1-1 Epidemiology of bacterial cystitis. The incidence of bacterial cystitis varies by age and sex. Women in their reproductive years are particularly prone to symptomatic episodes and account for the majority of visits to physicians in private offices and clinics. Approximately 20% of these women will experience recurrent urinary tract infections. Most recurrences are uncomplicated and can be managed by short courses of antibiotics or, if recurrences are frequent, by chronic suppression or postcoital antibiotics. The annual cost for the management of bacterial cystitis in the ambulatory care setting is estimated to be approximately $1 billion.

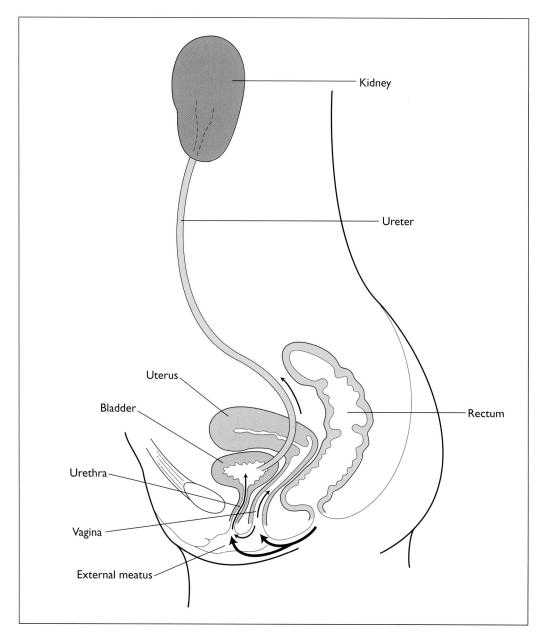

FIGURE 1-2 Pathogenesis of cystitis in women. Although bladder infections can result from the downward migration of organisms from an infected kidney, the overwhelming majority arise by ascent of pathogens from the rectum and vagina to the urethra meatus and bladder, leading to cystitis. If left untreated, the infection can further ascend to involve the kidneys (pyelonephritis). The rectum and vagina function as the reservoir of bacteria for sporadic infections, and unless potential pathogens are eradicated from these sources, they are also the reservoir for recurrent urinary tract infections. In men, the longer urethra is believed to protect against ascending infections.

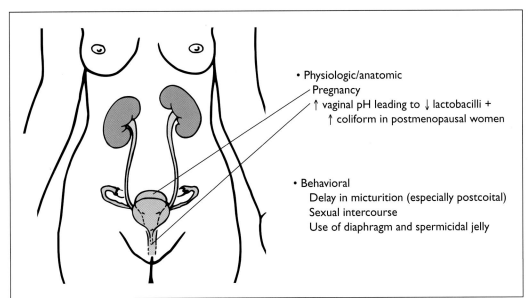

FIGURE 1-3 Risk factors for cystitis in women. Unique factors predisposing women to cystitis include behavioral and physiologic or anatomic ones. The higher risk of infection associated with pregnancy may be due to partial outlet obstruction brought on by the expanding uterus or from ureteral dilatation and the vesicoureteral reflux brought about by hormonal changes of pregnancy. Behavioral factors include delaying micturition, which leads to a higher residual volume and longer incubation time for the growth of bacteria. Sexual intercourse and the use of a diaphragm and spermicidal cream lead to vaginal colonization with potential uropathogens. The increased risk of cystitis found in postmenopausal women and women with bacterial vaginosis is believed to result from increases in vaginal pH, which decrease colonization with lactobacilli and promote colonization with coliform bacteria.

- Physiologic/anatomic
  - Pregnancy
    - ↑ vaginal pH leading to ↓ lactobacilli + ↑ coliform in postmenopausal women
- Behavioral
  - Delay in micturition (especially postcoital)
  - Sexual intercourse
  - Use of diaphragm and spermicidal jelly

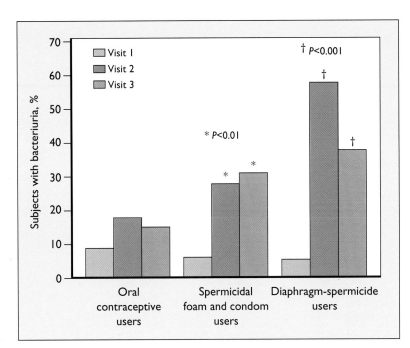

FIGURE 1-4 Effect of sexual intercourse and method of contraception on incidence of bacteriuria. In a study by Hooton and coworkers, women who used a spermicide (nonoxynol-9) with or without a diaphragm had a significantly higher risk of developing bacteriuria (> 10^2 colony-forming units of *Escherichia coli* per mL of urine) within 24 and 48 hours (visits 2 and 3) after intercourse than oral contraceptive users. Oral contraceptive users had only a marginal increase in the frequency of bacteriuria. Evidence from other studies, however, suggests that sexual intercourse itself is a contributing risk factor for urinary tract infections. (P = Values are derived from comparisons with the prevalence at visit 1.) (*Adapted from* Hooton *et al.* [1].)

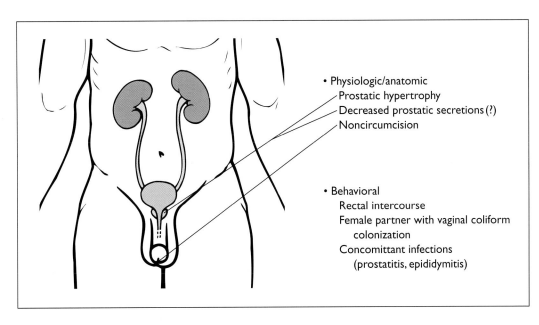

FIGURE 1-5 Risk factors for cystitis in men. Urinary tract infections are uncommon in men except at both ends of the age spectrum. Infections in young boys are often associated with congenital abnormalities in the renal tract. With older age, the enlarging prostate gland, reduced production of prostatic fluid (which may have antibacterial activity), and concomitant infections (prostatitis and epididymitis) all contribute to the increased frequency of urinary tract infections. Recently, two populations of young men have been identified to be at risk also: noncircumcised men and men who practice rectal intercourse. Noncircumcision leads to an increased risk of infection because of the enhanced bacterial colonization of the glans and prepuce. Rectal intercourse increases the risk through exposure to uropathogens in the anal canal.

- Physiologic/anatomic
  - Prostatic hypertrophy
  - Decreased prostatic secretions (?)
  - Noncircumcision
- Behavioral
  - Rectal intercourse
  - Female partner with vaginal coliform colonization
  - Concomittant infections (prostatitis, epididymitis)

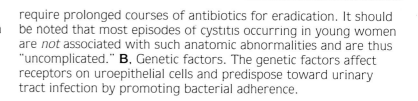

A. Common risk factors for cystitis in both sexes: Anatomic factors
Urethral stricture ↑ Residual volume ↓ Urinary flow Instrumentation Stasis ↓ Urinary acidification/concentration

B. Common risk factors for cystitis in both sexes: Genetic factors
Blood group B and AB who are nonsecretors of blood-group substances P1 blood group phenotype in patients without additional predisposing factors (vesicoureteral reflux) P2 blood group phenotype in adults Lewis blood group nonsecretor or recessive phenotypes

FIGURE 1-6 Common risk factors for cystitis in both sexes. **A,** Anatomic factors. Anatomic or physiologic risk factors common to both sexes include instrumentation or the presence of functional or anatomic abnormalities that alter urinary flow. The resultant infections are considered "complicated" in that they often recur, involve the upper renal tract (pyelonephritis), or require prolonged courses of antibiotics for eradication. It should be noted that most episodes of cystitis occurring in young women are *not* associated with such anatomic abnormalities and are thus "uncomplicated." **B,** Genetic factors. The genetic factors affect receptors on uroepithelial cells and predispose toward urinary tract infection by promoting bacterial adherence.

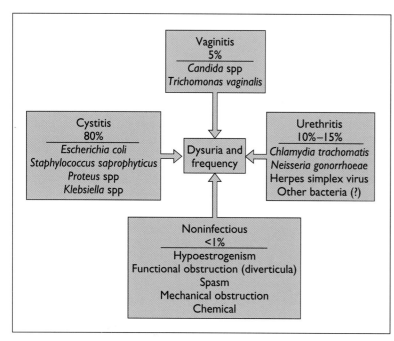

FIGURE 1-7 Causes of the acute dysuria–frequency syndrome. Symptoms of dysuria and frequency are nonspecific and can be caused by 1) classic cystitis with > 10^5 colony-forming units (cfu) of bacteria per mL of urine or low-count infection between 10^2 and 10^4 cfu/mL of urine; 2) urethritis by sexually transmitted disease agents; 3) vaginitis in which the resultant burning sensation may be described as "external" dysuria and vulvar irritation is also seen; and 4) noninfectious causes. Differentiation among these possible etiologies can be made from laboratory findings and further history.

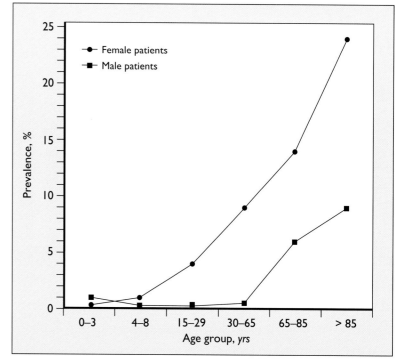

FIGURE 1-8 Prevalence of bacteriuria in the elderly. Approximately 20% of women and 3% of men in age group 65 to 70 years are affected by bacteriuria. By age 80, the prevalence of bacteriuria increases to 25% to 50% in women and to 20% in men. The possible reasons for the increased prevalence with advancing age include changes in bladder function, pelvic architecture, prostate size in men, more frequent instrumentation, bowel and bladder incontinence, waning immunologic status, and onset of concomitant debilitating illnesses.

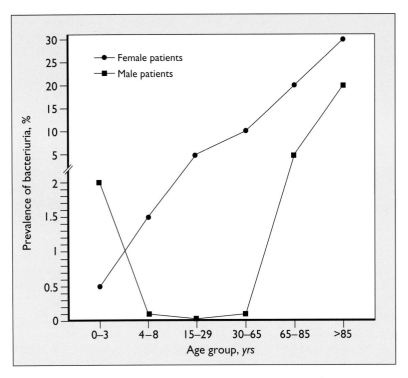

FIGURE 1-9 Lifetime frequency of bacteriuria. In children < 3 years of age, the frequency of urinary tract infections is higher for boys than girls. The occurrence of infection at this age often reflects underlying congenital abnormalities. During young adulthood, urinary tract infections are rare among men but quite common in women. In contrast to children, adult women with cystitis rarely have associated structural abnormalities. With advancing age, the prevalence of bacteriuria in both sexes increases, with women continuing to be at a greater risk (approximately 3:1 female-to-male ratio). Most of these episodes in both sexes are asymptomatic and transient, and they generally resolve without the need for specific antibiotic therapy.

BACTERIAL VIRULENCE FACTORS

Microbiology of uncomplicated cystitis	
Escherichia coli	80%
Staphylococcus saprophyticus	10%–15%
Klebsiella pneumoniae	3%
Proteus mirabilis	2%

FIGURE 1-10 Microbiology of uncomplicated cystitis. Greater than 95% of cases of uncomplicated cystitis are caused by a single bacterial species. In 80%, the responsible organism is *Escherichia coli. Staphylococcus saprophyticus* is the second most common uropathogen found among outpatient women. This organism is rarely found in nosocomial or catheter-associated urinary tract infections. The frequency of organisms from the *Enterobacteriaceae* family reflects the proximity of the rectum as a source and reservoir for bacteria that migrate toward the urethra, vagina, and bladder.

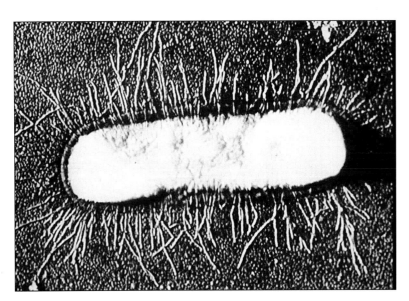

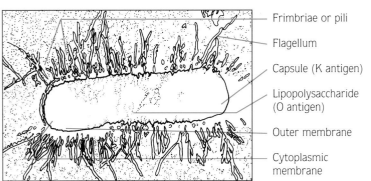

- Frimbriae or pili
- Flagellum
- Capsule (K antigen)
- Lipopolysaccharide (O antigen)
- Outer membrane
- Cytoplasmic membrane

FIGURE 1-11 Electron micrograph depicting the important components of the *Escherichia coli* bacterium. Pili or fimbriae mediate adherence to the uroepithelium. Capsular (K) polysaccharides coat the bacterium and protect it from phagocytosis and the complement-lysis system. The O capsular polysaccharides also protect the bacterium from serum bactericidal activity, and certain O polysaccharides (smooth type) appear to be more resistant to complement than others (rough strains). (*From* Duguid *et al.* [2]; with permission.)

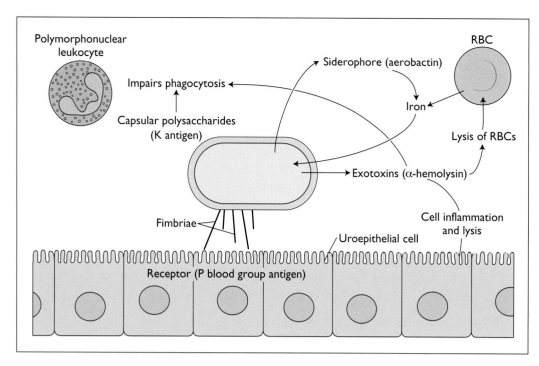

FIGURE 1-12 Interaction of bacterial virulence factors with host cell. Virulence factors interact in a complex manner. Fimbriae mediate attachment of the bacterium to uroepithelial cells, facilitating colonization and infection. Patients with certain P blood group antigens have receptors on their uroepithelial cells consisting of a Gal (α 1–4)Gal β terminal moiety that provides high-affinity attachment sites for *Escherichia coli* with P-fimbriae. These patients are more prone to recurrent infections, including pyelonephritis. The polysaccharide capsule is both antiphagocytic and anticomplementary. Other virulence factors include the elaboration of exotoxins (α-hemolysin), which mediate inflammation and cell lysis, and siderophores (aerobactin), which scavenge for iron necessary for bacterial growth. (RBC—red blood cell.)

Microbiology of complicated cystitis	
Escherichia coli	30%
Enterococci	20%
Pseudomonas spp	20%
Coagulase-negative staphylococci	15%
Klebsiella pneumoniae	5%
Proteus mirabilis	4%

FIGURE 1-13 Microbiology of complicated cystitis. The distribution frequency of pathogens causing complicated cystitis is listed. Compared with its role in uncomplicated cystitis, *Escherichia coli* is less prominent, although it is still the most common causative agent (30%) in complicated infections. Enterococci and *Pseudomonas* species increase in importance as uropathogens. Because complicated cystitis often recurs, the change in the pathogens is likely the result of selective antibiotic pressure from previous courses of antibiotics. Resistant organisms are more frequent.

DIAGNOSIS

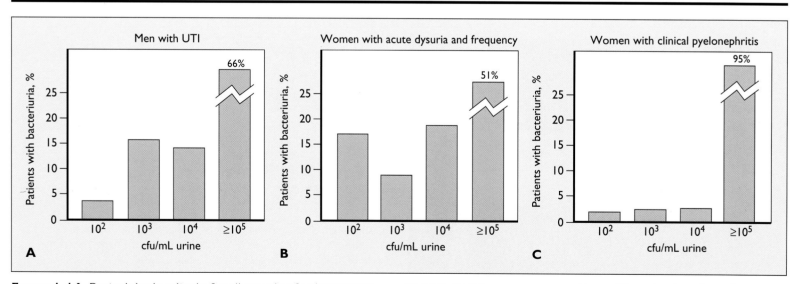

FIGURE 1-14 Bacteriologic criteria for diagnosis of urinary tract infection (UTI) from voided urine. **A**, Men with UTI. **B**, Women with acute dysuria and frequency. **C**, Women with clinical pyelonephritis. The most appropriate bacteriologic criteria for the diagnosis of UTI from voided urine specimens vary and depend on the population being studied. In 1956, Kass and colleagues [3] demonstrated that 95% of women with clinical pyelonephritis had urine cultures growing $\geq 10^5$ colony-forming units (cfu) per mL of urine (*panel 14C*), giving rise to the concept of "significant bacteriuria." In women presenting with acute dysuria and frequency who are unlikely to have pyelonephritis, Stamm and colleagues [4] showed that the traditional criterion of $\geq 10^5$ cfu/mL detected only 51% of lower tract infections, whereas a cutoff of $\geq 10^2$ cfu/mL had a diagnostic sensitivity of 0.95 and specificity of 0.85 (*panel 14B*). For men with UTI, Lipsky and colleagues [5] determined that $\geq 10^3$ cfu of one predominant organism had the best combination of sensitivity and specificity (0.97 and 0.97, respectively) (*panel 14A*).

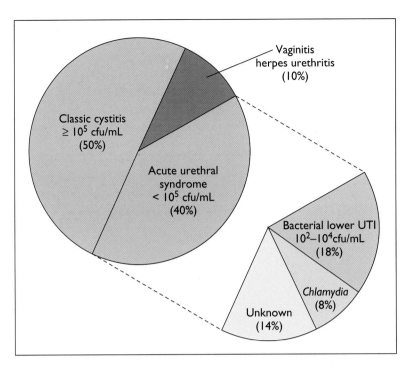

FIGURE 1-15 Relative frequencies of causes of acute onset of frequency/dysuria in young women. Half of the women who present with acute symptoms of dysuria and frequency have classic cystitis with $\geq 10^5$ colony-forming units (cfu) per mL on urine culture. Forty percent have $< 10^5$ cfu/mL of urine (acute urethral syndrome). Of this latter group, most (18%) have a urinary tract infection (UTI) with low counts of bacteria (10^2 to 10^4 cfu/mL of urine). Some (8%) have a urethral infection due to *Chlamydia*, the remainder (14%) have no identifiable causative agent [6].

Cystitis: Indications for pretreatment urine cultures

Culture indicated	Culture not indicated
Complicated infection	Uncomplicated infection
Persistent symptoms despite antibiotics	As "test of cure" (unless certain conditions are present—*eg*, pregnancy, in children, or obstructive uropathy)
Pregnancy	
Diabetes	
Recurrent infection	
Signs and symptoms of upper urinary tract infection (pyelonephritis)	

FIGURE 1-16 Indications for pretreatment urine cultures in cystitis. Empiric antibiotic therapy, without first obtaining a urine culture, is an acceptable cost-effective practice in women with uncomplicated cystitis. For women who are pregnant or diabetic, present with signs and symptoms of an upper urinary tract infection, or might otherwise have a complicated infection, urine cultures should be obtained before the start of antibiotics in order to identify antibiotic-resistant bacteria or a relapsing infection. Generally, test-of-cure urine cultures are not recommended at follow-up when patients have responded clinically to antimicrobial therapy. The exceptions are pregnant patients, children, or adults with obstructive uropathy, all of whom could suffer serious sequelae should infection persist.

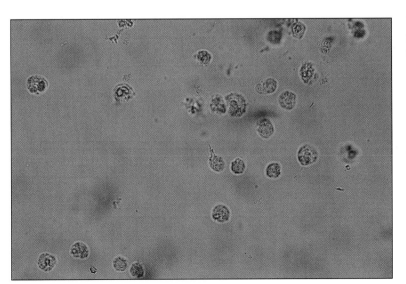

FIGURE 1-17 Light microscopy of unstained centrifuged urine showing pyuria and bacteriuria. The urine, a midvoid, clean-catched specimen, was centrifuged; the sediment re-suspended in urine; and a drop examined under a coverslip. Examination under high-dry magnification ($\times 400$) shows pyuria and bacteriuria. Both findings suggest the presence of a urinary tract infection. Finding at least one organism per high-power field when examining unstained, centrifuged urine under a light microscope has a sensitivity of approximately 93% (range, 91%–97%) and specificity of 77% (range, 50%–88%) when significant bacteriuria (*ie*, $\geq 10^5$ colony-forming units/mL of urine on culture), is used as the gold standard for diagnosis of infection [7].

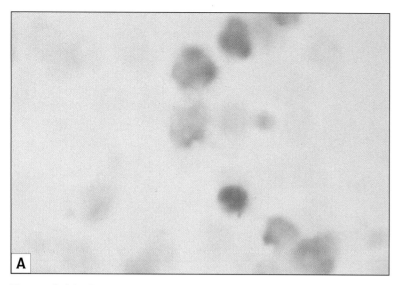

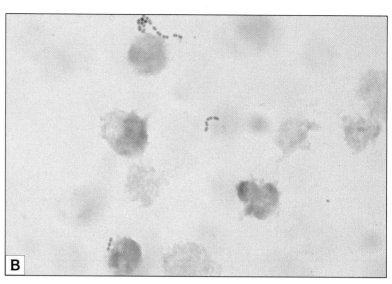

FIGURE 1-18 Gram-stained smears of urine from a patient with urinary tract infection. **A,** Uncentrifuged urine, examined under oil-immersion field ($\times$ 1000), shows leukocytes but no organisms, even though the patient has $\geq 10^5$ colony-forming units per mL of urine on culture. **B,** The same urine, when centrifuged before Gram staining, shows gram-positive bacteria (*Enterococcus*) in addition to leukocytes. Examination of uncentrifuged urine is commonly practiced but requires training and persistence ($\geq$ 5 fields/slide must be observed) to achieve high sensitivity. Centrifugation before Gram-staining improves sensitivity, and the results are more reproducible.

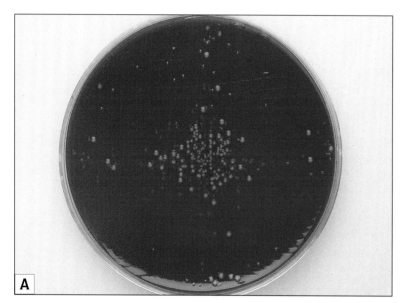

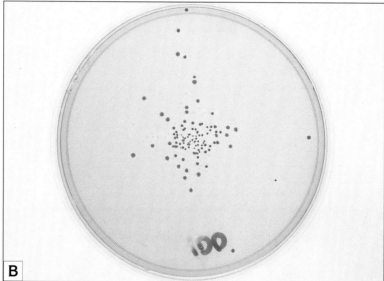

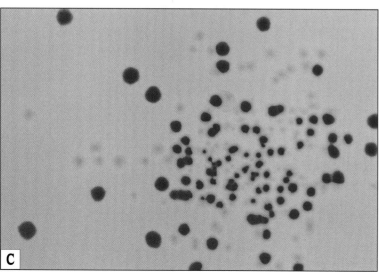

FIGURE 1-19 Urine cultures in urinary tract infection. **A,** Blood agar. **B,** MacConkey agar. **C,** Close-up of bacteria on MacConkey agar with backlighting. Urine is cultured quantitatively by inoculating 0.001 mL of urine, via a calibrated loop, onto a blood agar or MacConkey agar plate. The MacConkey agar is a selective medium that selectively inhibits the growth of gram-positive bacteria. The sole carbohydrate source in MacConkey is lactose, which also acts as an indicator. The close-up photograph with backlighting (*panel 19C*) shows two types of colonies: one that ferments lactose (*Escherichia coli*) and turns pink in this medium and a second colony type that does not ferment lactose and is colorless (*Pseudomonas aeruginosa*). Approximately 100 colonies of each type are seen on this plate, and thus, the culture will be reported quantitatively as $\geq 10^5$ colony-forming units per mL of urine.

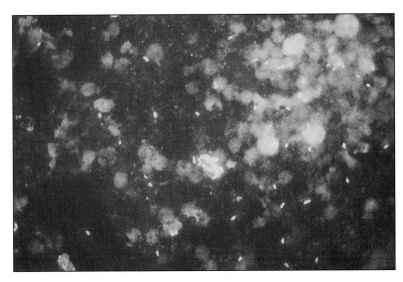

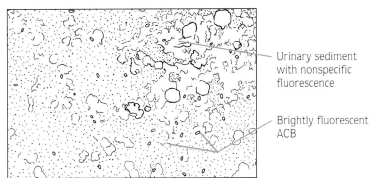

Urinary sediment with nonspecific fluorescence

Brightly fluorescent ACB

FIGURE 1-20 Fluorescein microscopy and the antibody-coated bacteria (ACB) assay in urinary tract infection (UTI). With the use of fluorescein-conjugated antihuman globulin, bacteria that are antibody-coated are brightly fluorescent when viewed under fluo-

rescein microscopy. The presence of five or more ACB under oil-immersion field ($\times$ 1000) constitutes a positive assay and is indicative of an upper UTI. Although the assay has been used successfully to localize the site of infection among women with outpatient UTI, false-positive results occur frequently in men with bacterial prostatitis, patients with indwelling urinary catheters, and patients with candiduria due to nonspecific binding of fluorescein-tagged immunoglobulin with yeasts. In these populations, the ACB assay has not proven to be useful [8].

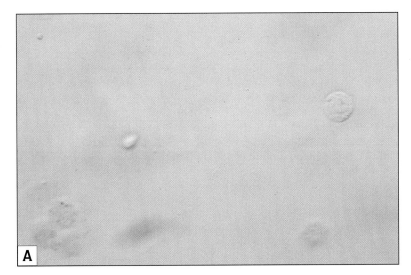

A

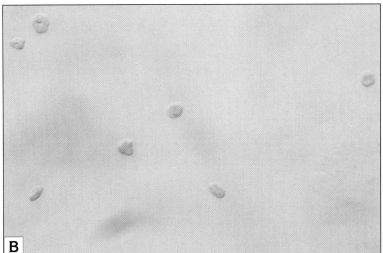

B

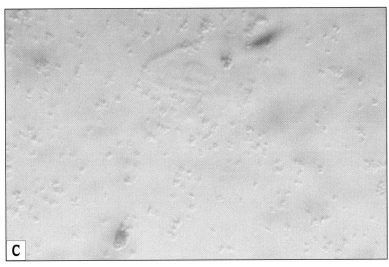

C

FIGURE 1-21 Urinalysis in the diagnosis of urinary tract infection. **A–C**, Wet-mount examination of midvoided, clean-catched urine showing pyuria (*panel 21A*), hematuria (*panel 21B*), and bacteri-uria (*panel 21C*). (*continued*)

D. Diagnostic significance of urinalysis and culture findings in urinary tract infection

	Pyuria	Hematuria	Bacteriuria	Culture $\geq 10^2$ cfu/mL
Classic cystitis	+++	++	+++	+++
Low-count infection	+++	+	+	+++
Urethritis	+++	+	+	+
Vaginitis	+	+	+	+

+++—usually; ++—sometimes; +—rarely.

cfu—colony-forming units.

FIGURE 1-21 (*continued*) **D,** Diagnostic significance of urinalysis and culture findings in urinary tract infection. Findings on low-power microscopic examination of urine, combined with urine culture, are helpful in differentiating the causes of acute, dysuria–urinary frequency syndrome. Patients with classic cystitis with significant bacteriuria ($\geq$ 105 colony-forming units [cfu] per mL of urine) will show pyuria and bacteriuria on urinalysis. Those having low-count infection with bacterial counts between 102 and 104 cfu/mL of urine will have pyuria but rarely bacteriuria on wet-mount examination [6]. Patients with urethritis have pyuria but not bacteria on urinalysis or urine culture. The urinalysis and urine culture in vaginitis are usually normal, but pyuria may reflect unrecognized trichomoniasis.

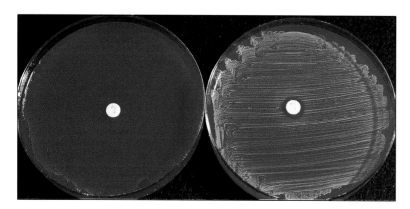

FIGURE 1-22 Culture for staphylococcal uropathogens using novobiocin susceptibility testing. Of the many staphylococci that are resistant to novobiocin, including *Staphylococcus saprophyticus, S. cohnii, S. xylosus, S. sciuri, S. lentus,* and *S. gallinarum,* only *S. saprophyticus* is clinically important as a uropathogen, causing up to 17% of outpatient urinary tract infections in women. A simple method to detect novobiocin-resistance is the disk diffusion procedure using a 5-µg novobiocin susceptibility disk on an agar plate streaked with staphylococci (0.5 McFarland suspension). Shown here are two urinary isolates of coagulase-negative staphylococci. The isolate on the right is novobiocin-resistant, as indicated by a zone diameter of < 16 mm, and therefore presumptively identified as *S. saprophyticus.*

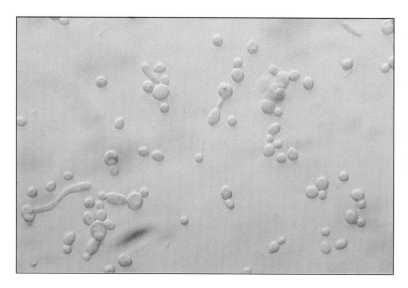

FIGURE 1-23 Urinalysis showing yeast forms in urinary tract infection. Examination of the centrifuged urine reveals yeast (both budding yeast and mycelial forms) and pyuria. Although candiduria is known to occur more frequently in patients recently treated with antibiotics, in diabetics, and in patients with indwelling Foley catheters, its clinical significance is uncertain—it may reflect colonization or infection with candidal cystitis or pyelonephritis. The colony count of *Candida,* the presence or absence of pyuria, and the presence or absence of mycelial forms all have been studied in an attempt to distinguish between colonization and infection, but they generally have poor discriminatory value [9].

CLINICAL FEATURES

Comparison of the clinical features of acute cystitis, urethritis, and vaginitis

Acute cystitis	Urethritis	Vaginitis
Internal dysuria	Internal dysuria	External dysuria
Frequency	Frequency (rare)	Vaginal discharge/odor
Urgency	Urgency (rare)	Vulvar irritation/pruritus
Cloudy urine	Vaginal discharge	Dyspareunia
Hematuria	Typical pathogens	Typical pathogens
Typical pathogens	*Chlamydia trachomatis*	*Candida albicans*
Suprapubic tenderness	*Neisseria gonorrhoeae*	*Trichomonas vaginalis*
Escherichia coli	*Herpes simplex*	
Staphylococcus saprophyticus		

FIGURE 1-24 Comparison of the clinical features of acute cystitis, urethritis, and vaginitis. The clinical presentation of acute cystitis, urethritis, and vaginitis can be similar, but there are distinguishing features. The dysuria experienced by patients with cystitis and urethritis is often described as internal or "deep-inside," whereas the localization of dysuria in vaginitis is more external and is likely to result from the passage of urine on an irritated or inflamed external genitalia. In addition, the symptoms of cystitis develop acutely. In contrast, the onset of symptoms associated with urethritis and vaginitis is often more gradual and generally milder. The presence of a vaginal discharge accompanying other symptoms of urethritis depends on the etiology and may result if the urethral pathogens are associated with cervicitis.

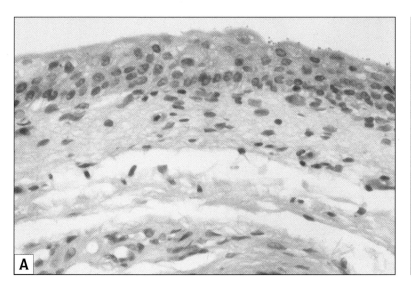

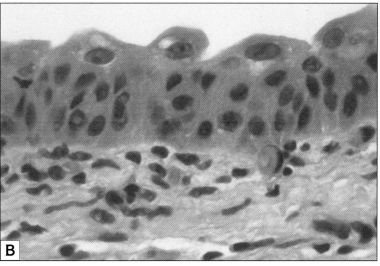

FIGURE 1-25 Histologic examination of normal bladder mucosa. **A**, Normal bladder mucosa (magnification, × 100) showing adherent streptococci on the luminal surface. There is no inflammatory infiltration of the mucosa or submucosa, suggesting that adherent microorganisms represent an early stage of infection or colonization. **B**, On higher-power examination (magnification, × 200), note the uniform nuclear size of mucosal cells and the larger outer layer of "umbrella" cells.

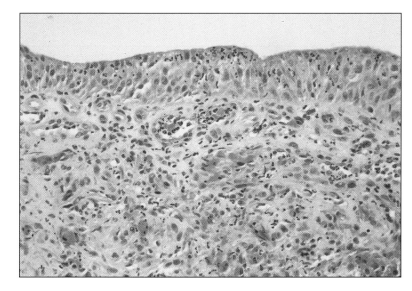

FIGURE 1-26 Histologic examination of bladder mucosa in acute cystitis. In acute cystitis, both the mucosa and submucosa are diffusely infiltrated with acute inflammatory cells (polymorphonuclear leukocytes). The lamina propria is edematous, and the capillaries are dilated and show leukocyte diapedesis. With severe acute cystitis, the urothelium can become hyperplastic and slough, resulting in mucosal denudation. (Magnification, × 50.)

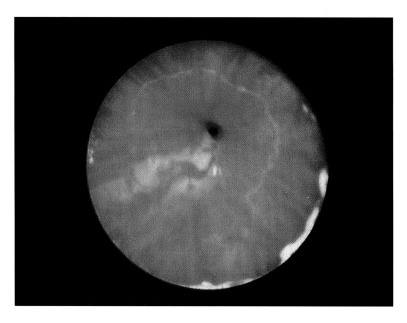

FIGURE 1-27 Acute urethritis seen with urethroscopy. Under urethroscopy, the urethra can be examined for signs of inflammation such as redness and exudate or pallor, atrophy, or friability, which can result from hypoestrogenism. In this figure, the redness and pus are characteristic of acute urethritis caused by either *Chlamydia trachomatis* or *Neisseria gonorrhoeae*. (*From* Scotti [10]; with permission.)

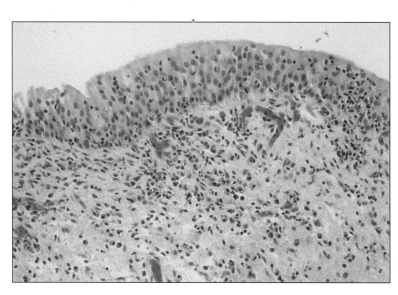

FIGURE 1-28 Histologic examination of bladder mucosa in chronic cystitis. In chronic cystitis, the mucosa and submucosa are edematous and infiltrated with mononuclear leukocytes. Both lymphocytes and plasma cells with cytoplasmic granules can be seen in the lamina propria. (Magnification, × 50.)

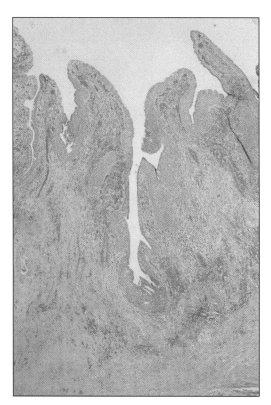

FIGURE 1-29 Histologic examination of bladder mucosa in chronic cystitis showing cobblestones and diverticuli. Chronic cystitis as a result of chronic outlet obstruction can lead to cobblestone and diverticuli formation in the bladder mucosa. Bladder wall biopsy from such an individual shows polypoid cystitis with hyperplastic bladder mucosa and edematous lamina propria resulting in the formation of broad and thin villous projections. The uroepithelium, although thickened, shows orderly maturation and should not be confused with papillary transitional cell carcinoma. The lamina propria contains chronic inflammatory cells. Not seen at this magnification is the muscular hyperplasia that is usually found.

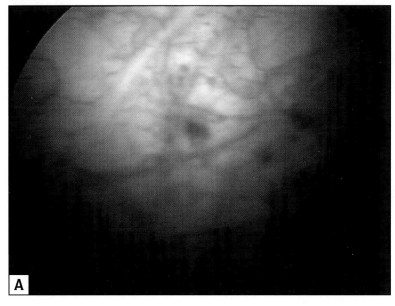 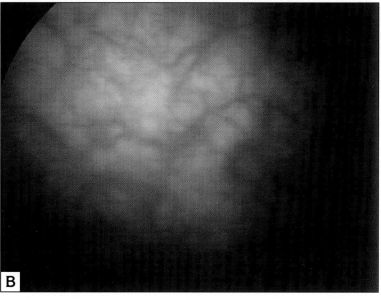

FIGURE 1-30 Cystoscopic views of bladder in interstitial cystitis. **A.** Cystoscopic view of bladder mucosa from a 29-year-old woman diagnosed clinically with interstitial cystitis. **B.** Cystoscopic view of normal bladder mucosa. The patient had complained of urinary frequency, pelvic pain, and vague bladder pressure for several years. Repeated urine cultures were negative for bacterial pathogens. Cystoscopy and hydrodilatation of this patient revealed petechial glomerulations that are consistent with her clinical diagnosis of interstitial cystitis. (*Courtesy of* J. McMurtry, MD.)

Characteristics of complicated versus uncomplicated urinary tract infections

Uncomplicated	Complicated
Female sex	Male sex
Young adults	Older age
Functionally and anatomically intact urinary tract	Functionally or anatomically abnormal urinary tract
Outpatient	Hospitalized
> 80% *Escherichia coli*	Broad range of pathogens
Antimicrobial resistance infrequent	Antibiotic resistance common
Oral therapy	Oral/parenteral therapies
Respond to short courses	Longer courses needed

FIGURE 1-31 Characteristics of complicated versus uncomplicated urinary tract infections (UTIs). Uncomplicated and complicated UTIs differ significantly in their underlying pathogenesis and their treatment. Uncomplicated infections occur most commonly in young adult women. They are not associated with abnormalities (either functional or anatomic) in the urinary tract and are generally caused by *Escherichia coli*. Complicated infections occur in both sexes. In fact, all UTIs in men should be considered complicated. Complicated infections are often associated with alterations in urinary flow or instrumentation or involve the upper urinary tract (pyelonephritis) and thus are prone to recur. Causative organisms in complicated infections are often antibiotic-resistant. As a result, treatment often requires extended-spectrum antibiotics or parenteral antibiotics, and longer courses are needed.

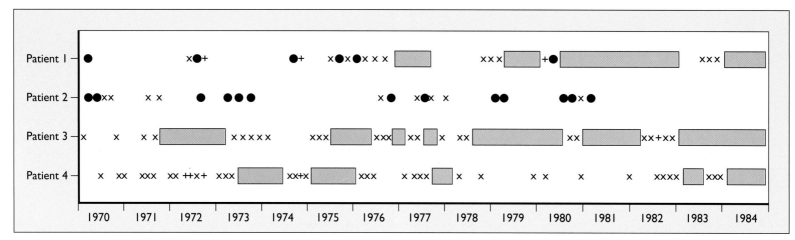

FIGURE 1-32 Patterns of recurrent urinary tract infections in four women. In this figure, the *solid circles* represent episodes of urethral syndrome, *crosses* acute cystitis, and *pluses* asymptomatic bacteriuria; *bars* indicate periods of antimicrobial prophylaxis. The natural history of recurrent urinary tract infections in women is marked by temporal clustering, with an average rate of 2.6 episodes per year (range, 0.3–7.6). Antimicrobial prophylaxis was highly effective in these women in preventing infectious episodes. The use of trimethoprim-sulfamethoxazole, however, was associated with the emergence of resistance in the past 5 years of the study. (*Adapted from* Stamm *et al.* [11].)

Recurrent urinary tract infections: Characteristics of reinfection versus relapse

	Reinfections	Relapse
Sex	Female	Male or female
Age	Young or middle-age	Premenarchal girls or older women
		Men or boys at any age
Type of infection	Uncomplicated	Complicated
Pattern of recurrence	Either infrequent with 1–2 episodes/yr or frequent with ≥ 3 episodes/yr	Recurrence within 1–2 wks after stopping antibiotics
Pathogen	Different pathogens or multiple strains involved	Identical pathogen causing prior infection
	Antibiotic resistance uncommon	Antibiotic resistance common

FIGURE 1-33 Characteristics of reinfection versus relapse of recurrent urinary tract infections. Reinfections occur in young adult or middle-aged women and generally appear in two patterns: either infrequently, with one to two episodes per year, or frequently, with multiple episodes per year (three to five episodes). Reinfections involve the lower urinary tract and therefore are largely uncomplicated. Although *Escherichia coli* may be repeatedly isolated, different strains are usually involved. Relapsing infections occur in both sexes generally in age groups different from those experiencing reinfections. Relapses usually reoccur within 1 to 2 weeks after stopping antibiotics. They are caused by the same organism responsible for the prior infection, suggesting a persistent nidus somewhere in the urinary tract (kidney in women, prostate or kidney in men). Relapsing infections are also often associated with antibiotic-resistant bacteria.

Predisposing factors for recurrent urinary tract infections

Reinfection	Relapse
Sexual intercourse	Functional or anatomic abnormality
Use of diaphragm and spermicide as contraceptives	Renal parenchymal infection (pyelonephritis) or bacterial prostatitis
Delay in micturition	Infected renal calculus
Genetic susceptibility (*eg,* nonsecretors of certain blood group substances)	Inadequate antibiotic treatment

FIGURE 1-34 Predisposing factors for recurrent urinary tract infections (UTIs). Relapsing UTIs are more likely to occur in the presence of functional or structural abnormalities of the urinary tract. They are also more likely to occur when a tissue focus of infection, *eg*, in the renal parenchyma or prostate, is involved. If antibiotic treatment is inadequate, infection persists and relapse occurs. Diagnostic work-up of relapses with ultrasonography, excretory urography or cystoscopy is indicated, especially if renal tract abnormalities are suspected. In contrast, reinfections are largely associated with behavioral factors. Genetic factors may play a role in increasing susceptibility to UTIs by promoting bacterial adherence and colonization at vaginal and periurethral sites. Because renal abnormalities are rarely found in reinfections, radiographic and urologic tests are generally not indicated.

TREATMENT

Treatment of uncomplicated cystitis

Antibiotic regimens	Comments
Single-dose antibiotics with TMP-SMX or quinolones	Less effective than multiple-day regimens
3-day regimens of TMP-SMX, TMP alone, fluoroquinolones, nitrofurantoin, β-lactam agents	Optimal balance between efficacy and side effects Fluoroquinolones are effective but expensive
7-day regimen of TMP-SMX, TMP, oral fluoroquinolones, β-lactam agents	Consider longer course in patients with diabetes, pregnancy, symptoms > 7 days, age > 65 yrs Longer regimens associated with more side effects

TMP-SMX—trimethoprim-sulfamethoxazole.

FIGURE 1-35 Treatment of uncomplicated cystitis. Uncomplicated cystitis can be managed by one of three strategies. Single-dose antibiotics is the most convenient method but is less effective than multiple-day regimens, in part because it does not reliably eradicate rectal and vaginal carriage. Single-dose β-lactam regimens have been particularly disappointing and should not be used. The 7-day regimen is the most effective but exposes the patient to the greatest amount of antibiotics and thus the most side effects. The 3-day regimen appears to be the optimal balance between efficacy and potential for side effects.

Comparative efficacy of antibiotics in the treatment of uncomplicated cystitis

Class of antibiotics	Comments
β-lactams	20%–30% of *Escherichia coli* are resistant to β-lactam antibiotics Ampicillin is less effective and has a higher recurrence rate compared with TMP-SMX
TMP-SMX	Considered drug of choice because of efficacy, low cost, and twice-daily dosing Sulfa component is responsible for side effects TMP alone may be as effective
Quinolones	Broad-spectrum of activity against gram-negative bacteria Effective and convenient dosing (twice-daily) Concerns of cost and risk of resistance (reserve for complicated urinary tract infection)

TMP-SMX—trimethoprim-sulfamethoxazole.

FIGURE 1-36 Comparative efficacy of antibiotics in the treatment of uncomplicated cystitis. The choice of antibiotics should be based on antimicrobial susceptibility of the organism and the patient's history (allergy). When the pathogen is unknown, the agent is chosen empirically. Ampicillin as an empiric choice is less than ideal, because currently 20% to 30% of *Escherichia coli* are resistant to it. Even when organisms are susceptible, ampicillin has a lower cure rate and higher recurrence rate when compared with treatment with trimethoprim-sulfamethoxazole [12]. Quinolone antibiotics exhibit broad-spectrum activity against most uropathogens and would be expected to be highly effective in the treatment of uncomplicated urinary tract infections. When cost is considered, however, trimethoprim-sulfamethoxazole must be considered the drug of choice in uncomplicated cystitis.

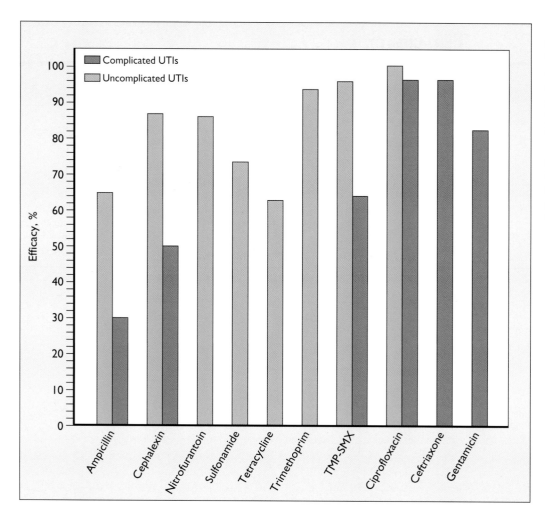

FIGURE 1-37 Expected efficacy of commonly prescribed antibiotics in the treatment of uncomplicated and complicated urinary tract infections (UTIs). The expected efficacy is based on antimicrobial susceptibility of commonly isolated uropathogens. For uncomplicated UTIs, the oral drugs trimethoprim-sulfamethoxazole (TMP-SMX), trimethoprim, and ciprofloxacin would be expected to have the highest cure rate (> 90%), whereas ciprofloxacin and the parenteral antibiotics ceftriaxone and gentamicin would be the most effective in complicated UTIs.

Treatment of complicated cystitis*	
Antibiotic regimens	**Comments**
Oral trimethoprim-sulfamethoxazole or fluoroquinolones for 7–14 days	For outpatient therapy of mild to moderate illness without nausea or vomiting

*Based on urine culture results.

FIGURE 1-38 Treatment of complicated cystitis. The treatment of complicated cystitis differs significantly from that of uncomplicated cystitis. Because of changes in antibiotic susceptibility and in the distribution of causative organisms, antibiotics with a more extended spectrum of activity against gram-negative bacteria, including *Pseudomonas*, are required. In addition, a longer duration of treatment is required because of the possibility of renal involvement (pyelonephritis). Patients with mild to moderate infection and those who can tolerate oral medications can be treated as outpatients with 7 to 14 days of oral trimethoprim-sulfamethoxazole or a quinolone. Severe constitutional symptoms imply systemic infection and generally require hospitalization and treatment with parenteral antibiotics (*see* Pyelonephritis).

Implications of complicated cystitis

Increased likelihood of urinary tract abnormality
Increased likelihood of occult pyelonephritis
Increased likelihood of resistant organisms
Pretreatment urine cultures essential
No single-dose antimicrobial therapy
Results of 3-day therapy unpredictable
Requires 7–14 days of antimicrobial therapy

FIGURE 1-39 Clinical and therapeutic implications of complicated cystitis. Complicated cystitis is often associated with a functional or anatomic abnormality of the renal tract, and the kidney may be involved (pyelonephritis). Pretreatment urine culture is indicated to identify the causative organism, especially if prior exposure to antibiotics might select for resistant strains. Short-course antibiotics (single-dose or 3-day therapy) are contraindicated because of low efficacy and risk of relapse.

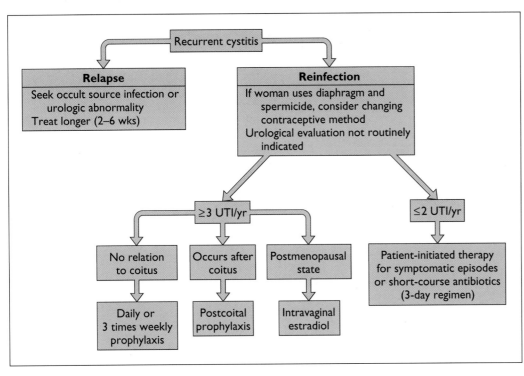

FIGURE 1-40 Approach to management of recurrent cystitis. The management of recurrent cystitis in women depends on whether the recurrent episode of infection is caused by the same uropathogen (relapse) or one different from that isolated from a prior episode (reinfection). Relapses are complicated infections, requiring longer courses of antibiotics for eradication (≥ 2 weeks of antibiotics). Reinfections occur in patients with normal urinary tracts, and therefore, urologic evaluations are not indicated routinely. The treatment options for recurrent uncomplicated cystitis depend on its frequency and underlying pathogenesis. Women with two or less episodes per year can be managed by patient-initiated single-dose antibiotics when symptoms occur or with short-course antibiotics (*eg*, 3-day regimen) on presentation to the physician. Women who suffer three or more reinfections per year are managed most cost-effectively by continuous or thrice-weekly antibiotic prophylaxis or, if their cystitis occurs after intercourse, by postcoital prophylaxis. Recurrent cystitis in post-menopausal women is related to altered vaginal flora with colonization by Enterobacteriaceae. Recurrent infections can be reduced by intravaginal administration of estriol [13]. (UTI—urinary tract infection.)

Indications for urologic studies in patients with urinary tract infections*	
Indicated	**Not indicated**
Failure to respond to appropriate antibiotics	Uncomplicated cystitis in young adult women
Relapsing infection	
Infection associated with obstructive uropathy	
Recurrent pyelonephritis	
Cystitis in children	
Cystitis in young adult men	

*Includes ultrasonography, excretory urography, cystoscopy, or computerized tomography.

FIGURE 1-41 Indications for urologic studies in patients with urinary tract infections. Most cystitis episodes occur in young women with normal urinary tracts. Urologic evaluations of this population will be of low yield, and therefore, they are generally not warranted. Diagnostic investigations, however, are indicated when the urinary tract infection fails to respond to appropriate antibiotics, when the infection relapses, when the infection involves the upper tract (pyelonephritis), when obstruction is found, or when structural or function abnormalities are suspected (*eg*, hematuria, infection in children and young adult men). In these settings, the likelihood of underlying functional or structural abnormality in the urinary tract is high, and urologic evaluation may lead to identification and surgical correction.

Management of bacteriuria in the elderly	
Asymptomatic	**Symptomatic**
Do not screen or treat because:	Treat with antimicrobial agents
Uncommonly leads to symptomatic infections	
Does not increase mortality	
Treatment does not lower mortality and may select for antibiotic-resistant organisms	

FIGURE 1-42 Management of bacteriuria in the elderly. Bacteriuria is common in elderly men and women. Management depends on whether the bacteriuria is symptomatic or not. When bacteriuria in the elderly is associated with urinary tract symptoms, it should be treated with antibiotics, just as a symptomatic infection at any age should be. Controversy had existed in the management of asymptomatic bacteriuria in the elderly, because early studies suggested that asymptomatic bacteriuria was associated with decreased survival. More recent evidence, however, suggests that asymptomatic bacteriuria neither increases mortality, nor does antimicrobial intervention lower the mortality rate [14]. Thus, current recommendations are to neither screen for or treat asymptomatic bacteriuria in the elderly.

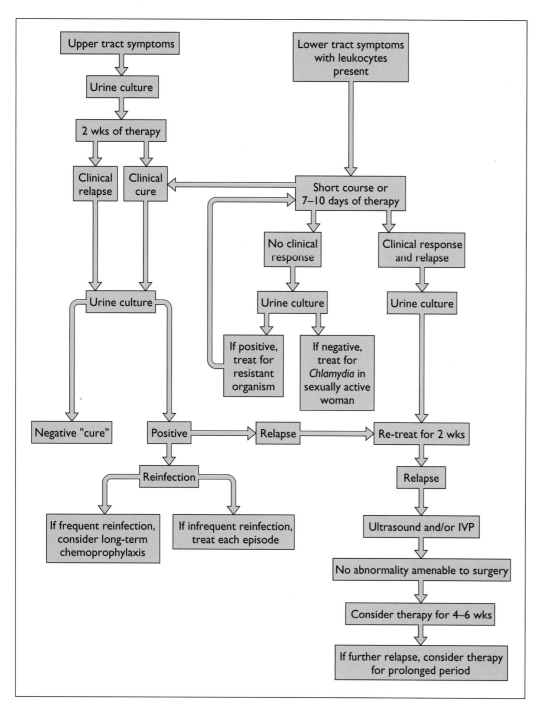

FIGURE 1-43 Algorithm for the management of patients presenting with upper and lower urinary tract symptoms. Initially, consider ultrasound and/or intravenous pyelogram (IVP) in all children and men with correction of significant lesions. Follow-up culture after cure is required only in pregnancy, in children, and in adults with obstructive uropathy. Consider ultrasound and/or IVP after three to four reinfections in women. (*Adapted from* Sobel and Kaye [15].)

References

1. Hooton TM, Hillier S, Johnson C, et al.: *Escherichia coli* bacteriuria and contraceptive method. *JAMA* 1991, 265:64–69.

2. Duguid JP, Smith IW, Dempster G, Edmunds PN: Nonflagella filamenta appendages ("fimbria") and hemagglutinating activity in *Bacterium coli*. *J Pathol Bacteriol* 1955, 70:335–349.

3. Kass EH, Finland M: Asymptomatic infections of the urinary tract. *Trans Assoc Am Physicians* 1956, 69:56–64.

4. Stamm WE, Counts GW, Running K, et al.: Diagnosis of coliform infection in acutely dysuric women. *N Eng J Med* 1982, 307:463–468.

5. Lipsky BA, Ireton RC, Fihn SD, et al.: Diagnosis of bacteria in men: Specimen collection and culture interpretation. *J Infect Dis* 1987, 155:847–854.

6. Stamm WE, Wagner KF, Amsel R, et al.: Causes of the urethral syndrome in women. *N Engl J Med* 1980, 303:409–415.

7. Jenkins RD, Fenn JP, Matsen JM: Review of urine microscopy for bacteriuria. *JAMA* 1986, 255:3397–3402.

8. Thomas V, Shelokov A, Forland M: Antibody-coated bacteria in the urine and the site of urinary tract infection. *N Engl J Med* 1974, 290:588–590.

9. Wong-Beringer A, Jacobs RA, Guglielmo J: Treatment of funguria. *JAMA* 1992, 267:2780–2785.

10. Scotti RJ: The urethral syndrome and urethral infections: I. Patient evaluation and infectious causes. *Infect Surg* 1989, 8:102–112.

11. Stamm WE, McKevitt M, Roberts PL, White NJ: Natural history of recurrent urinary tract infections in women. *Rev Infect Dis* 1991, 13:77–84.

12. Stamm WE, McKevitt M, Counts GW: Acute renal infection in women: Treatment with trimethoprim-sulfamethoxazole or ampicillin for two or six weeks: A randomized trial. *Ann Intern Med* 1987, 106:341–345.

13. Raz R, Stamm WE: A controlled trial of intravaginal estradiol in postmenopausal women with recurrent urinary tract infections. *N Engl J Med* 1993, 329:753–756.

14. Abrutyn E, Mossey J, Berlin JA, et al.: Does asymptomatic bacteriuria predict mortality and does antimicrobial treatment reduce mortality in elderly ambulatory women? *Ann Intern Med* 1994, 120:827–833.

15. Sobel JD, Kaye D: Urinary tract infections. *In* Mandell GL, Bennett JE, Dolin R (eds.): *Principles and Practice of Infection Diseases*. New York: Churchill-Livingstone; 1995:662–690.

Selected Bibliography

Abrutyn E, Mossey J, Berlin JA, et al.: Does asymptomatic bacteriuria predict mortality and does antimicrobial treatment reduce mortality in elderly ambulatory women? *Ann Intern Med* 1994, 120:827–833.

Hooton TM, Hillier S, Johnson C, et al.: *Escherichia coli* bacteriuria and contraceptive method. *JAMA* 1991, 265:64–69.

Jenkins RD, Fenn JP, Matsen JM: Review of urine microscopy for bacteriuria. *JAMA* 1986, 255:3397–3402.

Johnson JR: Virulence factors in *Escherichia coli* urinary tract infections. *Clin Microbiol Rev* 1991, 4:80–128.

Stamm WE, Hooton TM: Management of urinary tract infections in adults. *N Engl J Med* 1993, 329:1328–1334.

CHAPTER 2

Pyelonephritis

Michel G. Bergeron
Dominique Giroux
Claude Delage

THE NORMAL KIDNEY

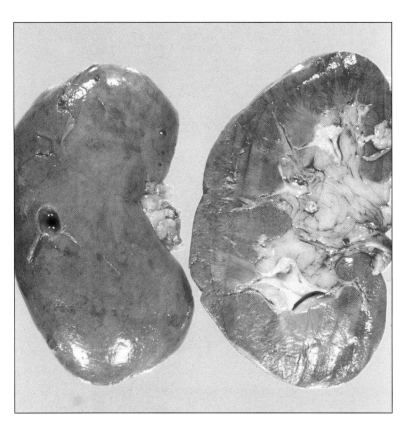

FIGURE 2-1 Gross photograph of a normal kidney. A normal kidney is seen with a cyst on its surface, a common finding on autopsy.

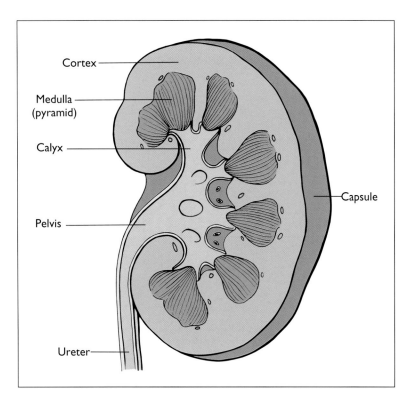

FIGURE 2-2 Histology of the normal kidney.

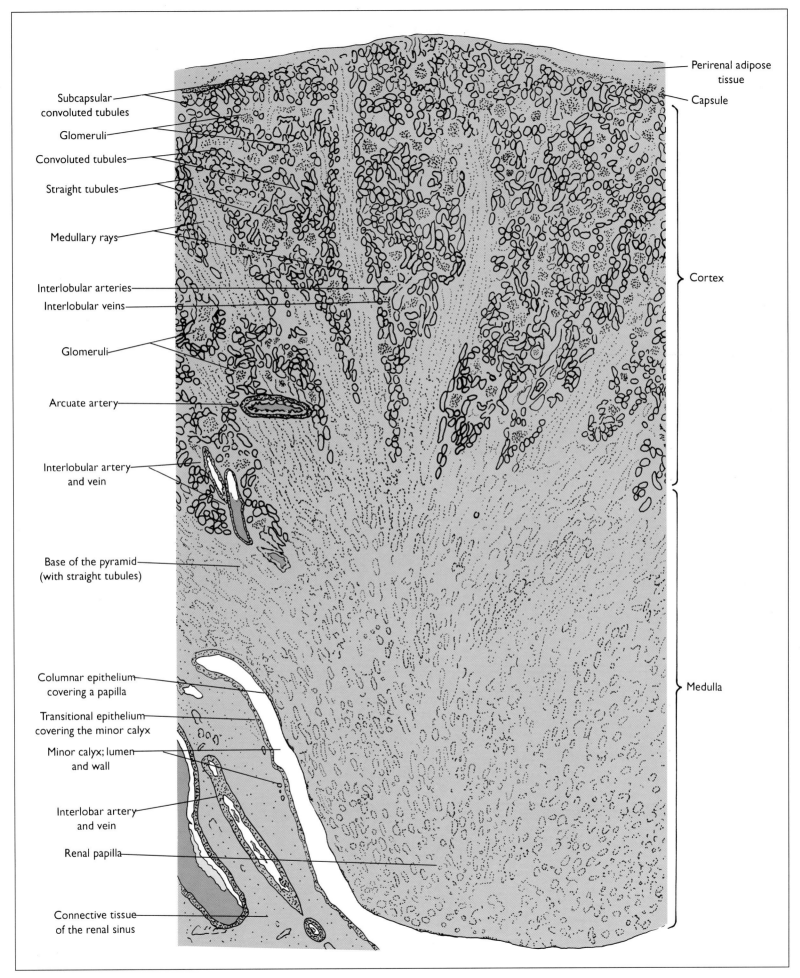

Perirenal adipose tissue

Capsule

Subcapsular convoluted tubules

Glomeruli

Convoluted tubules

Straight tubules

Medullary rays

Cortex

Interlobular arteries

Interlobular veins

Glomeruli

Arcuate artery

Interlobular artery and vein

Base of the pyramid (with straight tubules)

Medulla

Columnar epithelium covering a papilla

Transitional epithelium covering the minor calyx

Minor calyx; lumen and wall

Interlobar artery and vein

Renal papilla

Connective tissue of the renal sinus

FIGURE 2-3 Cross-sectional anatomy of a normal kidney showing the cortex, medulla, and renal papilla. (*Adapted from* Eroschenko [1].)

PATHOGENESIS

Normal host defenses against pyelonephritis: Bladder and ureter

Bladder level	Regular emptying of the bladder
	Urine characteristics: low pH, hyperosmolality, and urea content are deterrent to bacterial growth
	Tamm-Horsfall protein prevents binding of mannose-sensitive strains of *Escherichia coli*
	Natural vesicoureteral barrier
Ureter level	Natural flow of urine down the ureter to the bladder
	Peristaltic movement of the ureter

FIGURE 2-4 Normal host defenses against pyelonephritis: Bladder and ureter. At the bladder level: To invade the upper urinary tract, bacteria have to cross several barriers and evade local defenses that protect the kidney against infection. One of the most effective barriers is the normal flushing mechanism of the bladder, which prevents the establishment of bacteria in the bladder. Normally, unless the vesicoureteral sphincter is incompetent, or urine does not reflux into the ureter, so even in the presence of cystitis, bacteria have no access to the kidney. Urine by itself, although not bactericidal, does not favor bacterial growth. Tamm-Horsfall protein is secreted by cells of the ascending loop of Henle and reaches the urine in high concentration. It may prevent colonization and the establishment of cystitis by *Escherichia coli* expressing type 1 and S fimbriae. At the ureter level: The natural flow of urine and the peristaltic movement of the ureter are two important mechanisms that limit the ascent of pathogens moving upstream. Only selected bacteria with important adhesive properties can reach the kidney.

Normal host defenses against pyelonephritis: Kidney

Cellular defense: macrophages, endothelial cells, tubular cells, polymorphonuclear cells

Cytokines produced by these cells: tumor necrosis factor, IL-1, IL-2, IL-6, IL-10, interferon-α

Mediators of inflammation: leukotrienes, thromboxanes, prostacyclin, prostaglandins, platelet-activating factor

Nitric oxide

Antibody response: IgM, IgA, IgG

IL—interleukin.

FIGURE 2-5 Normal host defenses against pyelonephritis: The kidney. The host–pathogen interaction in the kidney is extremely complex, and the roles played by the different components of the cellular and humoral response are not well understood. Once bacteria have reached the papillary and medullary regions, they start to multiply, and several host cell lines, including macrophages, endothelial cells, tubular cells, and polymorphonuclear cells, are activated. As infection progresses, many cytokines are produced, as well as mediators of inflammation including nitric oxide, which favors vasodilatation and migration of cells at the site of infection. The exaggerated inflammatory response that is observed in severe pyelonephritis seems to contribute to renal damage.

Host defenses against pyelonephritis: The medulla facilitates bacterial invasion

10,000 times less bacteria are needed to infect the medulla than the cortex

Ammonia, found in high concentration in the medulla, may inactivate complement

High osmolality, low pH, and limited blood flow in the medulla limit chemotaxis of polymorphonuclear cells

FIGURE 2-6 Host defenses against pyelonephritis: The medulla facilitates bacterial invasion. The fact that host defenses in the medullary region of the kidney are limited generally favors the pathogen, explaining why the medulla is the primary site where bacteria can easily establish themselves.

Host defenses against pyelonephritis: Humoral immunity

Role poorly understood
IgM, IgG antibodies in serum/urine follow pyelonephritis
Protective role of immunoglobulins controversial
Vaccine development in experimental animals

FIGURE 2-7 Host defenses against pyelonephritis: Humoral immunity. The role of humoral immunity is also complex and poorly understood. It is known that the production of IgM antibody is observed only in the first episode of pyelonephritis. IgG antibody to lipid A (a major and potent component of endotoxins of Enterobacteriaceae) seems also to correlate with major kidney damage, suggesting that endotoxin may play a determinant role in the pathogenesis of pyelonephritis. In animal models, the protective role of specific antibodies to O and K antigens and to fimbrial antigens has been demonstrated, but in humans, their role is unclear.

Virulence factors of uropathogenic bacteria in pyelonephritis: K antigen and adhesions

Pathogenic factors	Role
K antigen	Protects against phagocytosis
Fimbrial adhesins P fimbriae (MR) S fimbriae (MR) Nonfimbrial adhesins F adhesins	MR fimbriae, including P and S fimbriae and F adhesins, seem necessary for *Escherichia coli* to reach pelvis and renal parenchyma P fimbriae block phagocytosis

MR—mannose-resistant.

FIGURE 2-8 Virulence factors of uropathogenic bacteria in pyelonephritis: K antigen and adhesins. Depending on their virulence factors, especially their adhesive properties, bacteria invade either the low or upper urinary tract. For example, *Escherichia coli* from pyelonephritis patients adhere better to uroepithelial cells than *E. coli* cystitis isolates or nonpathogenic *E. coli* isolated from feces. These adhesins are in general fimbrial in nature and are encoded in genes found on the chromosomes. P fimbriae that are associated with pyelonephritis bind to glycoprotein receptors (gal–gal), which, although observed throughout the uroepithelium, are mainly concentrated in the kidney. The binding of *E. coli* to these receptors is not inhibited by mannose and is called *mannose-resistant*, in contrast to mannose-sensitive binding observed in lower urinary tract infection strains. The role of fimbriae has also been demonstrated in *Proteus mirabilis* and *Klebsiella* species.

Virulence factors of uropathogenic bacteria in pyelonephritis: Other factors

Pathogenic factors	Role
Motility (gram-negative)	Ascend the ureter against flow of urine
Endotoxins (gram-negative)	Decrease ureteral peristalsis Increase kidney inflammatory response
Urease (*Proteus*)	Increase capacity to induce pyelonephritis
Hemolysin	Better invasion and tissue damage
Aerobactin	Siderophore that increases iron uptake and virulence (iron is an essential nutrient of bacteria)

FIGURE 2-9 Virulence factors of uropathogenic bacteria in pyelonephritis: Other factors. Invasion of the kidney by bacterial pathogens is a sequential process in which several virulence factors, including fimbrial and nonfimbrial adhesins and their intrinsic motility, allow microbes to reach the kidney. Once at the site of infection, especially the medulla, which is more susceptible to gram-negative pathogens, specific virulence factors, including endotoxin, urease, hemolysins, aerobactins, K antigens, and P fimbriae, either stimulate an exaggerated host response or reduce the killing capacity of cellular defenses. In complicated pyelonephritis, in which natural host defenses are impaired, less virulent pathogens may also induce this disease.

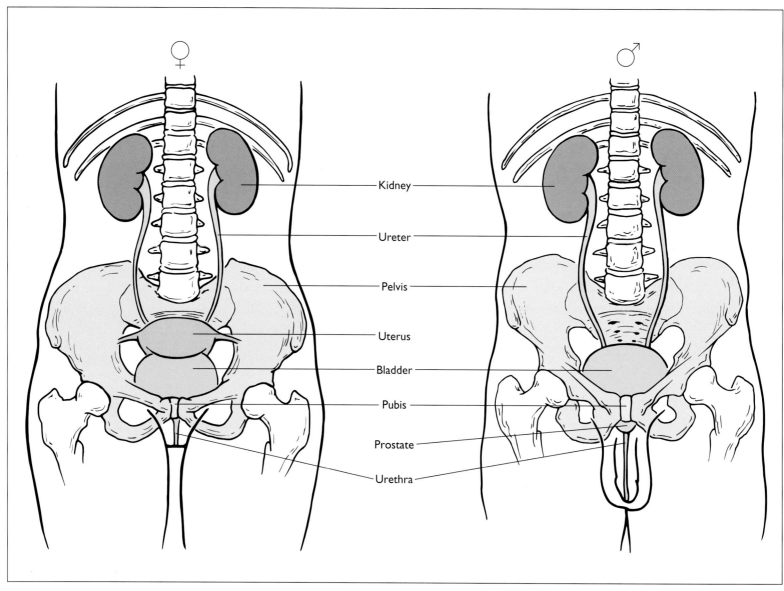

FIGURE 2-10 Anatomy of the normal male and female urinary tracts. Pyelonephritis is almost exclusively an ascending infection in which bacteria progress from the bladder to kidney parenchyma. In normal humans, urine flows down from the kidney to the ureter and bladder, but urine usually does not flow back from the bladder to the ureter, because there is a very effective sphincter at the vesicoureteral junction. Uropathogenic bacteria in the urine, their endotoxins, and/or the local inflammatory response of the bladder contribute to the breakdown of the vesicoureteral barrier, which leads to vesicoureteral reflux and allows bacteria to move up the ureter.

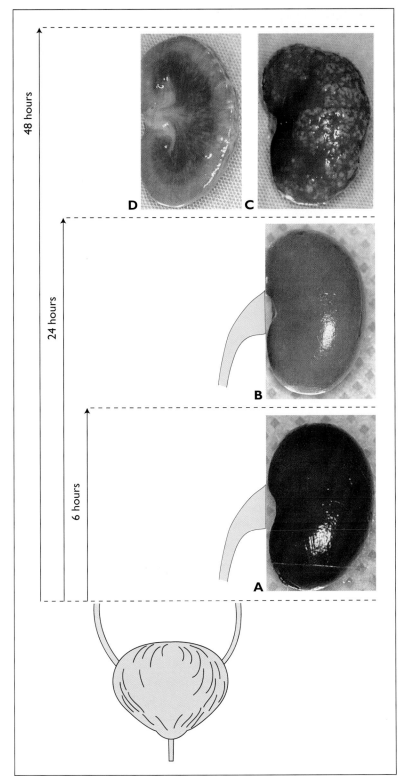

FIGURE 2-11 Serial rat kidneys showing progress of ascending pyelonephritis after induction with a uropathogenic strain of *Escherichia coli*. In ascending pyelonephritis, once bacteria break through the vesicoureteral barrier, it takes approximately 6 hours to reach the collecting proximal and distal tubules. Up to that time, the macroscopic and histologic appearances of the kidney are perfectly normal, and the number of colony-forming units (cfu) of *E. coli* is low (*A*). In the papilla, counts may reach between 10^1 to 10^3 cfu/g of tissue, whereas in the medulla and cortex the bacteria are usually undetectable at this early stage of disease. By 24 hours, even though bacteria multiply and double their population every 20 minutes, the tubular epithelium is still normal, but the kidney is edematous and pale (*B*). Bacterial endotoxin or other toxins released locally activate macrophages and other cells (endothelial, lymphocytes, kidney cells), which release different proinflammatory cytokines. Nitric oxide also contributes to this initial pallor and is associated with vasoconstriction and limited circulation to the renal parenchyma. This anoxia is the prelude to further damage, as it favors bacterial growth. By 48 hours, the bacteria are growing extremely rapidly and counts of $\geq 10^5$ cfu/g of tissues are observed. Polymorphonuclear cells infiltrate the tubules, damaging the tubular cells, and there is marked edema of the kidney. In the transverse section of the kidney (*D*), the cortical region is pale and edematous with multiple abscesses, whereas the medullary region is inflamed and highly vascularized and the papilla swollen. On the surface of the kidney (*C*), multiple abscesses are present. Irregular swelling is also evident.

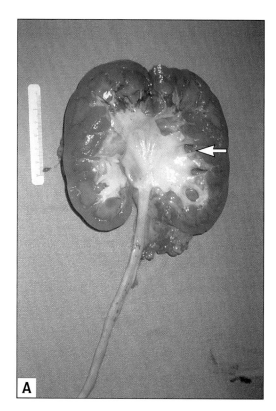

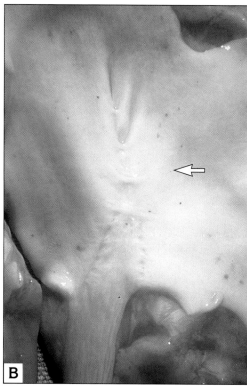

A **B**

FIGURE 2-12 Gross pathologic changes seen in kidney in acute pyelonephritis. Uncomplicated pyelonephritis occurs mainly in women. It presents itself as four major syndromes: subclinical pyelonephritis, moderate or severe acute pyelonephritis, pyelonephritis in pregnant women, and recurrent pyelonephritis. In men, some consider that all pyelonephritis should be classified as complicated, but some men, usually under age 60 with no apparent focus of infection in the prostate, can be classified as having uncomplicated pyelonephritis, which can be moderate or severe. **A** and **B**, Scar tissue (*arrows*) at the ureteropyelic region of the kidney, which could possibly be associated with silent or moderate recurrent pyelonephritis. As can be seen, the kidney was apparently normal.

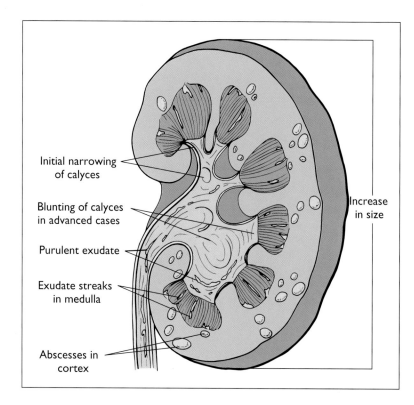

Initial narrowing of calyces

Blunting of calyces in advanced cases

Purulent exudate

Exudate streaks in medulla

Abscesses in cortex

Increase in size

FIGURE 2-13 Diagram of the histopathologic changes observed in the kidney in acute pyelonephritis. In uncomplicated acute pyelonephritis, the bacterial invasion and degree of renal damage are limited. The infection is probably limited to the pyelocalyceal-medullary region, involving focal areas. In severe uncomplicated acute pyelonephritis, the inflammation is probably more severe than in subclinical and acute pyelonephritis and likely covers a larger area of the kidney. As infection progresses, the bacteria can invade the bloodstream and induce septicemia, which may be associated with septic shock. Kidney infection rarely impairs renal function in adults, unless there are major predisposing factors, including obstruction of the urinary flow and diabetes, or if renal function is already altered by the underlying diseases. In children with anatomic or physiologic dysfunction, pyelonephritis may be associated with severe renal impairment. Proper antibiotics and release of obstruction on most occasions restore the "normal" structure of the kidney.

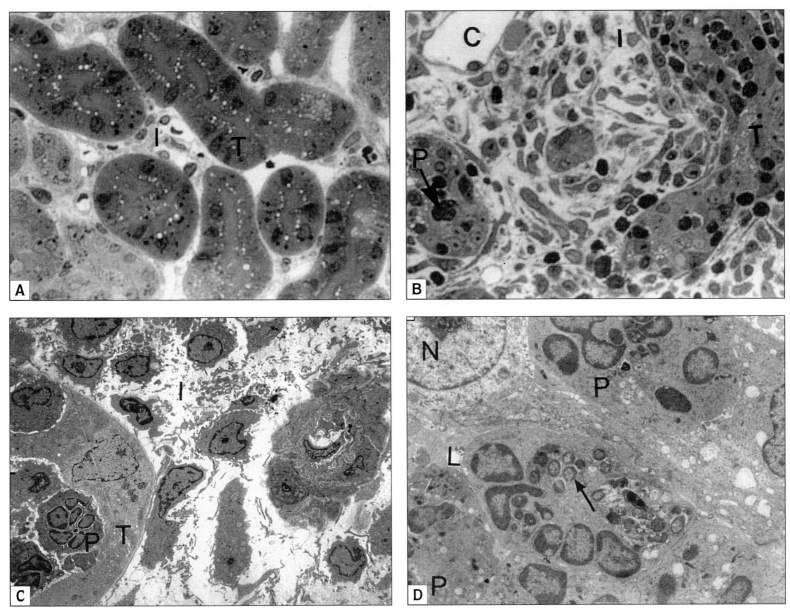

FIGURE 2-14 Histologic changes observed in severe pyelonephritis. The presence of bacteria in the tubules and renal parenchyma during pyelonephritis induces a marked local cellular and humoral response. Inflammatory cells migrate into the interstitium under chemotactic stimuli and then release free oxygen radicals and lysosomal enzymes into their environment. Although these products are essential for bacterial killing, they are in part responsible for deleterious effects to host cells, including tissue damage and scar formation, with the ensuing altered renal function and permanent kidney damage. **A,** Light microscopy of normal kidney. (Original magnification, × 1800.) **B,** Light microscopy of infected kidney. There is marked edema of the interstitial space and abundant inflammatory cells within tubular lumen and interstitium seen in this view of experimental pyelonephritis. (Original magnification, × 1800.) **C,** Electron microscopic studies showing marked cellular invasion and edema of the interstitium and numerous polymorphonuclear cells (PMNs) in the tubular lumen in experimental pyelonephritis. (Original magnification, × 3500.) **D,** Electron microscopic studies showing PMN invasion of tubular lumen and tubular cells. Numerous *Escherichia coli* (*arrow*) can be seen within PMNs in the tubular lumen in experimental pyelonephritis. (C—capillaries; I—interstitial space; L—lumen; N—nucleus of tubular cells; P—PMN; T—tubules.) (Panels 14A, 14B, and 14D *from* Tardif *et al.* [2]; with permission.)

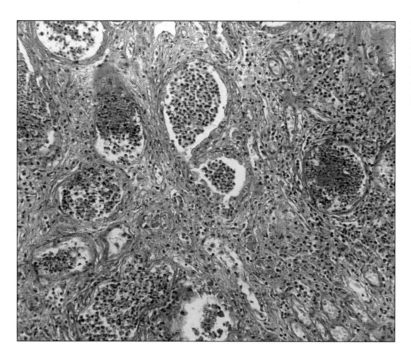

FIGURE 2-15 Histopathologic examination of kidney in acute pyelonephritis. A light microscopic view of human kidney shows massive infiltration of the tubular lumen and interstitial space by inflammatory cells consisting mainly of polymorphonuclear cells with a number of lymphocytes and plasma cells. (Hematoxylin-eosin stain; original magnification, × 250.)

MICROBIOLOGY AND ETIOLOGY

Microbiology in pyelonephritis	
Uncomplicated	**Complicated**
Escherichia coli (≥ 80%)	*Escherichia coli* (± 50%)
Proteus mirabilis	*Klebsiella* spp
Klebsiella pneumoniae	*Proteus* spp
Staphylococcus saprophyticus	*Pseudomonas* spp
Staphylococcus epidermidis	*Serratia* spp
	Enterobacter spp
	Enterococcus spp
	Staphylococcus spp
	Yeast

FIGURE 2-16 Microbiology in pyelonephritis. *Escherichia coli* is the most common cause of uncomplicated and complicated pyelonephritis, but the relative frequency of other pathogens increases in complicated pyelonephritis and varies depending on the underlying pathology or abnormality. Although pyelonephritis is generally caused by one pathogen, multiple bacteria may be isolated when structural abnormalities are present. Microorganisms observed in complicated infections are more a reflection of hospital flora. *Corynebacterium* group D2 and cell-wall deficient bacteria have also been observed rarely in patients with pyelonephritis [3].

Gram-Negative Bacteria

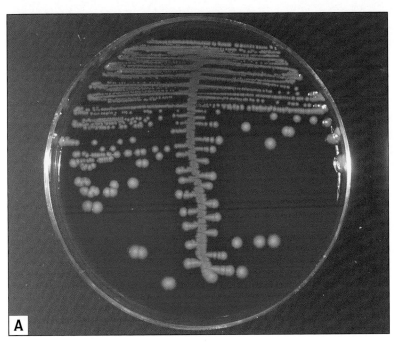

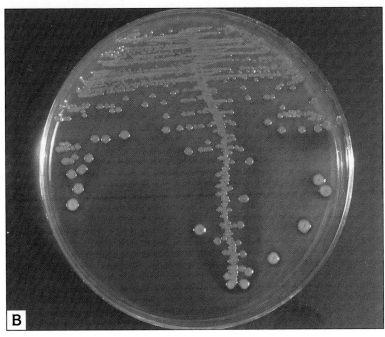

FIGURE 2-17 Culture plates with *Escherichia coli* colonies. *E. coli* is responsible for > 80% of uncomplicated pyelonephritis, whereas it is responsible for 50% of cases of complicated pyelonephritis. The uropathogenic strains have fimbriae that facilitate their attachment to uroepithelial cells. They may produce hemolysins that probably induce renal injury and bacterial persistence. **A,** On blood agar, large colonies of *E. coli,* 1 to 3 mm in diameter, appear glistening and are low convex in shape. **B,** On MacConkey agar, *E. coli* appears as pink colonies (rapid lactose fermenters) that may be surrounded by a red and opaque zone of precipitated bile coming from the media.

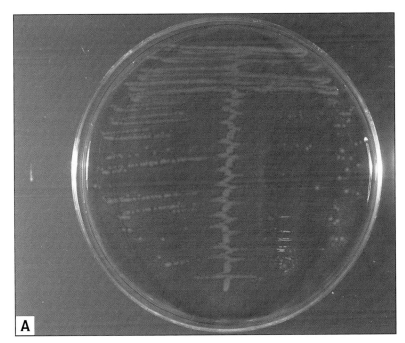

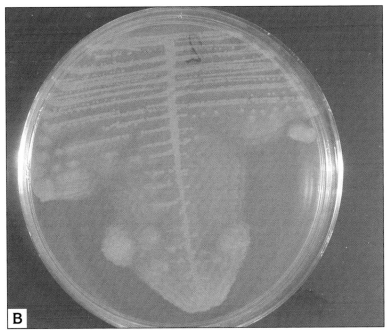

FIGURE 2-18 Culture plates showing *Proteus* colonies. *P. mirabilis,* like *Klebsiella pneumoniae,* can cause both uncomplicated and complicated pyelonephritis, whereas other *Proteus* species are more often associated with complicated pyelonephritis. **A,** On blood agar, *Proteus* produces swarming colonies, spreading a grayish-blue uniform film all over the media surface. This migration occurs in periodic cycles, producing concentric zones. **B,** On MacConkey agar, uncolored (nonlactose-fermenters) and swarming colonies can be observed.

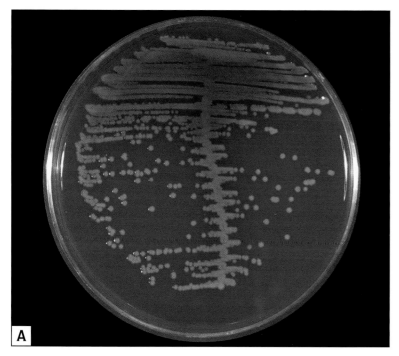
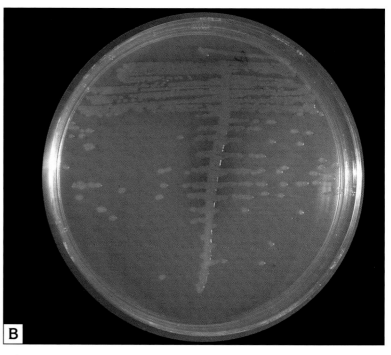

FIGURE 2-19 Culture plates showing *Pseudomonas* colonies. *Pseudomonas*, *Serratia*, *Proteus* (other than *P. mirabilis*), enterococci, many staphylococci, and yeast are often associated with complicated pyelonephritis. **A**, On blood agar, *Pseudomonas* produces flat or low convex colonies, 2 to 4 mm in diameter. A number of colony types may occur: smooth, coliform, rough, mucoid, gelatinous, and dwarf. A blue pigment is observed due to the production of pyocyanin. **B**, On MacConkey agar, *Pseudomonas* appears as colorless colonies, although pigmentation can also be observed.

Gram-Positive Bacteria

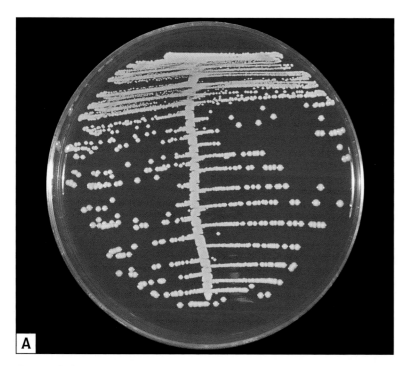
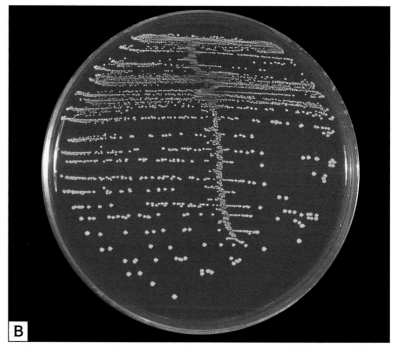

FIGURE 2-20 *Staphylococcus* colonies on blood agar. **A**, *Staphylococcus saprophyticus* colonies on blood agar. Colonies are slightly convex with a slight yellow tint. *S. saprophyticus* is resistant to novobiocin (5 µg), whereas other *Staphylococcus* are susceptible. **B**, *Staphylococcus epidermidis* colonies on blood agar. Colonies are smooth, circular, and opaque with a white pigment. No hemolysis is produced.

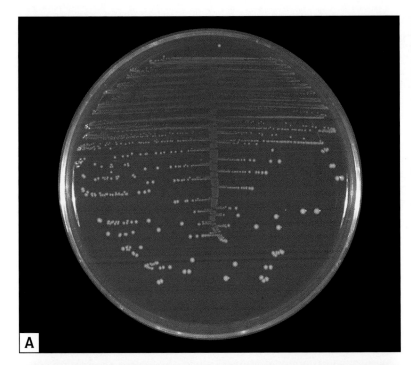

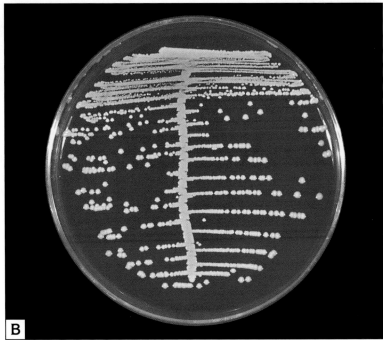

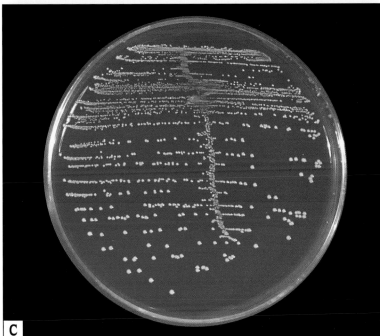

FIGURE 2-21 *Enterococcus* colonies on blood agar. **A,** *Enterococcus* produces translucent colonies that are white to grayish and less opaque than *Staphylococcus epidermidis* colonies (*panel 21C*). Differentiation of *Enterococcus* from *Staphylococcus* is done with the catalase test: *Staphylococcus* is catalase-positive, *Enterococcus* is catalase-negative. *Enterococcus'* capacity to grow in 6.5% sodium chloride broth and on bile-esculine agar and its ability to hydrolyze esculine are commonly used to distinguish the enterococci from other streptococci. **B,** *S. saprophyticus.* **C,** *S. epidermidis.*

CLINICAL SYNDROMES

Clinical presentations of uncomplicated pyelonephritis

Women	Subclinical (silent) pyelonephritis
	Acute pyelonephritis
	(moderate/severe)
	Pyelonephritis in pregnancy
	Recurrent pyelonephritis
Men	Acute pyelonephritis
(aged < 60 years)	(subclinical/moderate/severe)

FIGURE 2-22 Clinical presentations of uncomplicated pyelonephritis. In women, there are four major syndromes of uncomplicated pyelonephritis: subclinical, acute (which will be managed differently depending on whether it is moderate or severe), pyelonephritis in pregnancy, and recurrent. In men, whether all urinary tract infections should be classified as complicated pyelonephritis is still controversial, but some men, usually under age 60 who have no apparent focus of infection in the prostate, can be classified and treated as having uncomplicated pyelonephritis. Pyelonephritis in these men can be subclinical, moderate, or severe.

Complicated pyelonephritis

Occurs in men and women (often elderly)
Associated with underlying disorder:
  Structural or functional abnormalities
    Obstruction
    Calculi
    Neurologic diseases
    Vesicoureteral reflux
    Impaired renal functions
  Urologic manipulations
    Drainage devices/urinary catheter
    Urinary instrumentation
    Renal transplantation
  Underlying diseases
    Diabetes
    Immunosuppressed or immunodeficient host
    Sickle cell traits
    Cystic renal disease

FIGURE 2-23 Complicated pyelonephritis. In both men and women, complicated pyelonephritis is generally the result of structural and functional abnormalities, urologic manipulation, or underlying disease, which reduce the host's response or increase his or her susceptibility to infection. In men, pyelonephritis with a prostatic focus of infection as well as recurrent pyelonephritis are considered complicated. Pyelonephritis in the elderly may also be considered complicated [3].

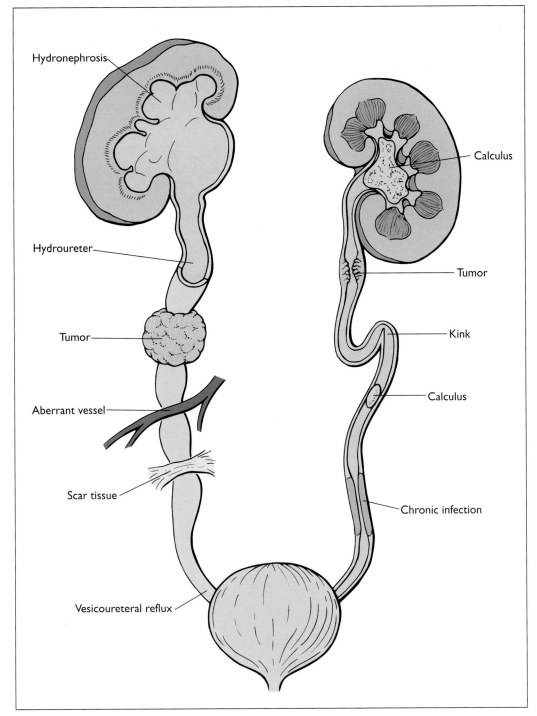

Hydronephrosis

Hydroureter

Tumor

Aberrant vessel

Scar tissue

Vesicoureteral reflux

Calculus

Tumor

Kink

Calculus

Chronic infection

Figure 2-24 Diagram of the underlying structural and functional abnormalities that define complicated pyelonephritis.

Clinical features of acute pyelonephritis

Few symptoms
Fever
Chills, rigors
Flank pain
Nausea, vomiting
Renal angle tenderness
Associated symptoms of concurrent cystitis/prostatitis

Figure 2-25 Clinical features of acute pyelonephritis. On examination, the kidney may or may not be tender on palpation. Occasionally, patients will have right upper-quadrant pain, mimicking acute cholecystitis, or pain radiating from the back to the inguinal region, simulating renal stones. Moreover, symptoms of both cystitis and pyelonephritis may resolve spontaneously without therapy. If pyelonephritis does not respond to adequate therapy or occurs in men, one should suspect obstruction caused by a urologic abnormality or renal stones. In patients with acute pyelonephritis, the physical examination rarely reveals bilateral tender and swollen kidneys, although imaging studies often disclose bilateral lesions.

Clinical features of subclinical (silent) uncomplicated pyelonephritis

Silent pyelonephritis frequently occurs in patients presenting with lower urinary tract symptoms (*eg*, frequency, dysuria, burning on micturition)

FIGURE 2-26 Clinical features of subclinical (silent) uncomplicated pyelonephritis. A major problem in diagnosing pyelonephritis is that up to 30% of women in primary-care settings and up to 80% of indigent patients seen in emergency rooms suffering from clinically apparent cystitis also have silent, invasive bacterial infections of the renal parenchyma. This infection is indistinguishable from lower urinary tract infection (UTI), because most patients have dysuria and pyuria but no back pain. The presence of antibody-coated bacteria in the urine used to diagnose this entity is debatable. Subclinical pyelonephritis resolves rapidly with antibiotic therapy, but a high percentage of patients relapse following short-term treatment and even after a week or two of "appropriate" therapy. Subclinical pyelonephritis is more common in pregnant women with UTI, patients who had a previous UTI before age 12 years, and those who had previous pyelonephritis or more than three UTIs in the past year.

DIAGNOSIS

Laboratory diagnosis of pyelonephritis

Urinalysis
Leukocyte esterases
Nitrate reduction
Proteinuria
Gram stain of urine (gram-positive vs gram-negative)
Midstream urine culture
Blood culture
Sedimentation rate
C-reactive protein
Antibody-coated bacteria (if subclinical pyelonephritis suspected)

FIGURE 2-27 Laboratory diagnosis of pyelonephritis. Following a direct microscopic examination of midstream urine to check for pyuria (≥ 10 leukocytes/mm^3), Gram stain should be done on all urine of patients with suspected pyelonephritis. A Gram stain on urine culture, which must be requested specifically from the laboratory, will allow the immediate distinction between gram-negative and gram-positive pathogens, for which therapy is considerably different. Nitrate reduction can also reveal the presence of bacteria, but false-negative tests are common. Urine culture, in general, will reveal $\geq 10^5$ bacteria/mL of urine. Erythrocyte sedimentation rate and C-reactive protein can be elevated but are not specific, and blood culture may be positive in $\geq 25\%$ of cases of acute severe pyelonephritis.

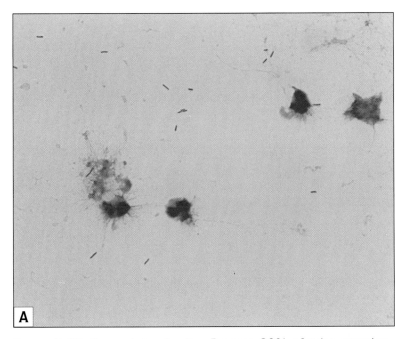

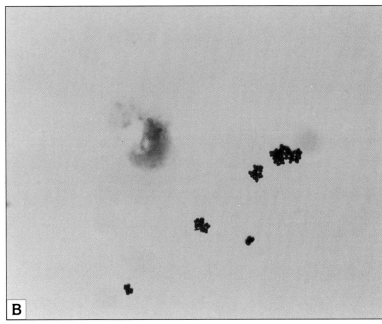

FIGURE 2-28 Gram stain of urine. Because 80% of urine samples that reach the microbiology laboratory are negative, most microbiologists do not do a Gram stain on urine. In pyelonephritis, the physician should ask specifically the laboratory to do a Gram stain, because it is crucial that the initial medication be oriented toward gram-positive or gram-negative bacteria. **A,** Gram-negative bacilli in urine with polymorphonuclear cells. **B,** Gram-positive cocci in urine.

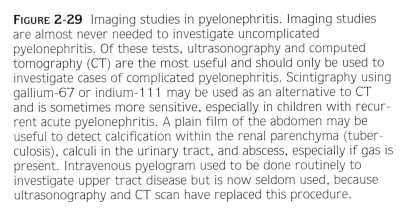

Imaging studies in pyelonephritis

Flat-plate radiograph of abdomen
Ultrasonography
Scintigraphy
Computed tomography
Magnetic resonance
Intravenous pyelography

FIGURE 2-29 Imaging studies in pyelonephritis. Imaging studies are almost never needed to investigate uncomplicated pyelonephritis. Of these tests, ultrasonography and computed tomography (CT) are the most useful and should only be used to investigate cases of complicated pyelonephritis. Scintigraphy using gallium-67 or indium-111 may be used as an alternative to CT and is sometimes more sensitive, especially in children with recurrent acute pyelonephritis. A plain film of the abdomen may be useful to detect calcification within the renal parenchyma (tuberculosis), calculi in the urinary tract, and abscess, especially if gas is present. Intravenous pyelogram used to be done routinely to investigate upper tract disease but is now seldom used, because ultrasonography and CT scan have replaced this procedure.

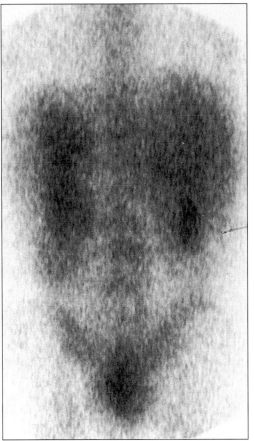

FIGURE 2-30 Renal gallium-67 scan in a young girl with bilateral acute pyelonephritis. There is great uptake in both kidneys due to the inflammation in this child with recurrent acute pyelonephritis. There is no uptake of isotope in normal kidneys. Isotope studies are rarely needed to investigate pyelonephritis but may be useful in cases in which pyelonephritis is suspected but ultrasound and computed tomography studies are negative, or when computed tomography scans are not available. It may also be useful to distinguish between an inflammatory and noninflammatory renal mass detected by other radiologic means. It is more often used in children than in adults.

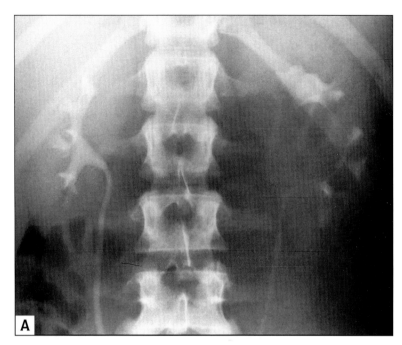

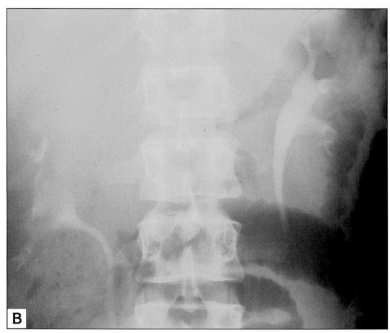

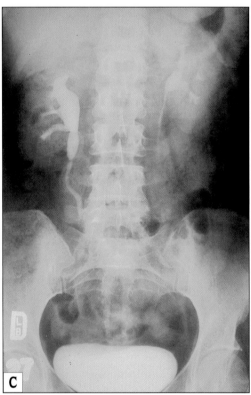

FIGURE 2-31 Intravenous pyelography in acute noncomplicated bacterial pyelonephritis. In 75% of cases, there are no changes on intravenous pyelogram. **A**, In 20% of cases, there may be a global or focal enlargement, as seen here in the left kidney. **B**, An impaired excretion or delayed appearance time, as well as decreased contrast density may also be a sign of pyelonephritis, as seen in the right kidney. **C**, Decreased filling, nonhomogeneous filling, attenuation of the collecting system, mucosal edema, poor definition of renal margins, and pyeloureteral dilatation occur in a very limited number of cases.

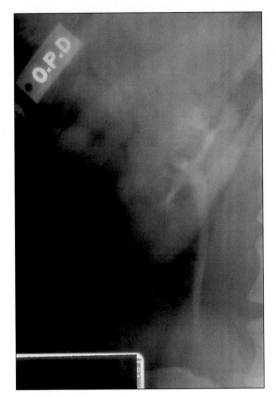

Imaging abnormalities in pyelonephritis

Clinical syndromes	Ultrasound	Computed tomography
Silent or acute moderate pyelonephritis	No lesion	No lesion or very limited lesion
Acute severe pyelonephritis	Renal enlargement (40%–90%)	Wedged-shaped lesions, (> 90%)
Complicated pyelonephritis	Renal enlargement (≈ 90%) Hypoechoic lesion (≈ 50%)	Focal or multifocal masslike lesion (> 90%)

FIGURE 2-33 Imaging abnormalities in pyelonephritis [4,5].

FIGURE 2-32 Intravenous pyelogram showing renocortical atrophy in complicated pyelonephritis. Intravenous pyelogram can show irregular atrophy of the cortical region, distension of the calyces (drumstick), general atrophy of the affected kidney with compensatory contralateral hypertrophy, and hypertrophy of the unaffected region of the infected kidney.

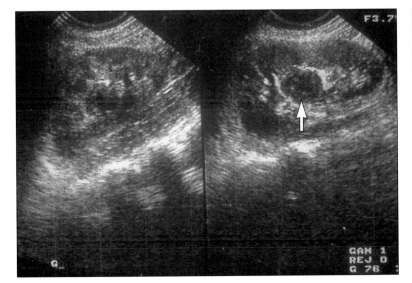

FIGURE 2-34 Ultrasound imaging in acute pyelonephritis. Ultrasound has the advantages of being rapid, noninvasive, relatively inexpensive, and accessible, and there is no exposure to radiation. It has now replaced intravenous pyelogram as the first means of evaluation of uncomplicated and complicated pyelonephritis. In acute pyelonephritis, the kidney shows renal enlargement, and in complicated pyelonephritis, hypoechoic lesions (*arrow*) may be observed. Ultrasound can detect abscesses of ≥ 2 cm in size and gas. Ultrasound is extremely useful for the confirmation of pyelonephritis during pregnancy and may be used to detect lower urinary tract obstruction and the presence of residual urine.

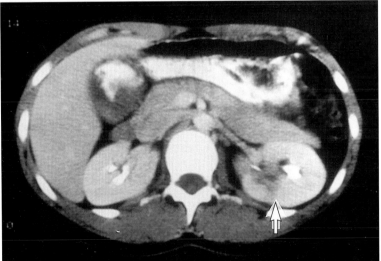

FIGURE 2-35 Computed tomography in acute pyelonephritis. On computed tomography scan, the masslike lesion of pyelonephritis is often well defined, because it is less dense than the cortex. It can be irregular with a nonhomogeneous center (*arrow*), as seen on the left kidney. The contralateral kidney is normal.

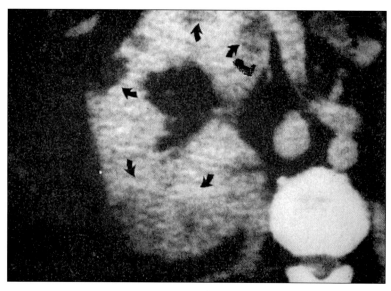

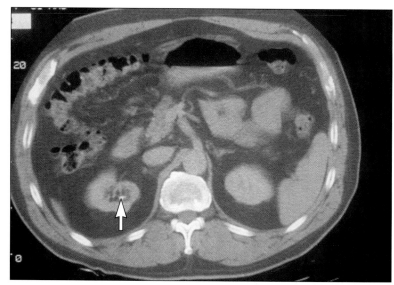

FIGURE 2-36 Computed tomography in acute pyelonephritis showing multifocal and diffuse masslike lesions (*arrows*). They often disappear after therapy. (*From* Huang [6]; with permission.)

FIGURE 2-37 Computed tomography (CT) scan showing renal atrophy in acute pyelonephritis. The CT scan shows irregular surface (atrophy) of the right kidney (seen on the left side), as compared with the left kidney, and distended calyces (*arrow*). Although CT is extremely sensitive to define intra- and perirenal suppuration, it is not as effective as intravenous pyelogram to detect abnormalities of the collecting system. Wedged-shaped lesions are seen in > 90% of patients with acute uncomplicated pyelonephritis. Focal and multifocal masslike lesions have also been observed in > 90% of patients with complicated pyelonephritis. Because intravenous pyelogram requires the administration of contrast material, it should thus be reserved for patients in whom ultrasonography is negative. Magnetic resonance imaging offers no advantages over CT scan.

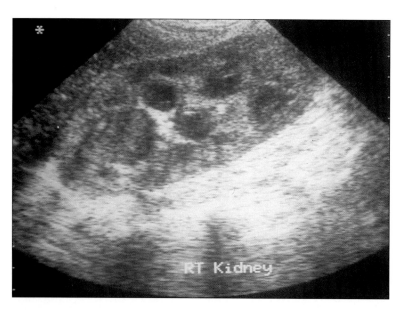

FIGURE 2-38 Ultrasound showing pyonephrosis. Echography demonstrates the presence of hydronephrosis and echogenic content on collecting system. A stone and/or a mass in the retroperitoneum usually will be causing the obstruction. A computed tomography scan usually is not necessary, unless a tumor is suspected. For pyonephrosis, nephrostomy is recommended, even though a nephrectomy is necessary in a high percentage of cases, because it diminishes morbidity and mortality.

COMPLICATIONS

Complications of pyelonephritis

Bacteremia/septicemia
Sepsis/disseminated intravascular coagulation
Septic shock
Local complications
  Pyonephrosis
  Microabscesses
  Intrarenal abscess
  Perinephric abscess
  Necrotizing papillitis
Chronic (persistent) pyelonephritis
Rejection of transplanted kidney

FIGURE 2-39 Complications of pyelonephritis. Both complicated and uncomplicated pyelonephritis can be associated, in both men and women, with gram-negative septicemia, which may induce septic shock. A borderline or low blood pressure associated with symptoms of urinary tract infection should suggest the possibility of septicemia. Pyonephrosis, microabscess, perinephritic abscess, and intrarenal abscess are usually not observed following uncomplicated pyelonephritis but are the results of renal infection associated with structural or functional abnormalities, urologic manipulations, and underlying diseases.

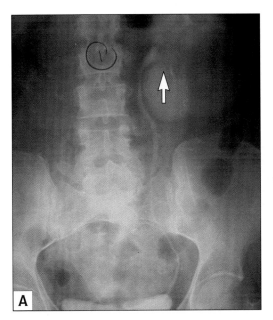

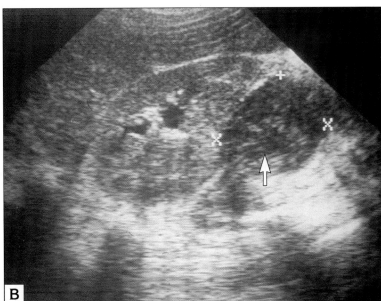

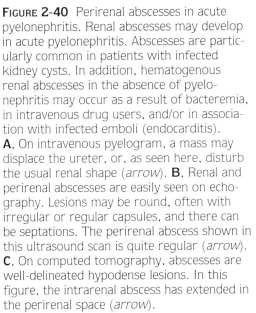

FIGURE 2-40 Perirenal abscesses in acute pyelonephritis. Renal abscesses may develop in acute pyelonephritis. Abscesses are particularly common in patients with infected kidney cysts. In addition, hematogenous renal abscesses in the absence of pyelonephritis may occur as a result of bacteremia, in intravenous drug users, and/or in association with infected emboli (endocarditis).
A, On intravenous pyelogram, a mass may displace the ureter, or, as seen here, disturb the usual renal shape (*arrow*). **B**, Renal and perirenal abscesses are easily seen on echography. Lesions may be round, often with irregular or regular capsules, and there can be septations. The perirenal abscess shown in this ultrasound scan is quite regular (*arrow*).
C, On computed tomography, abscesses are well-delineated hypodense lesions. In this figure, the intrarenal abscess has extended in the perirenal space (*arrow*).

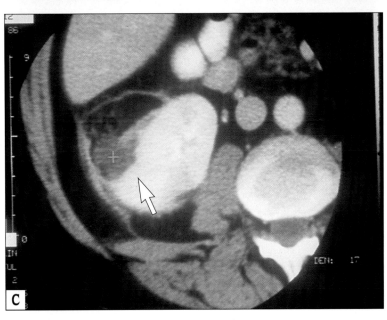

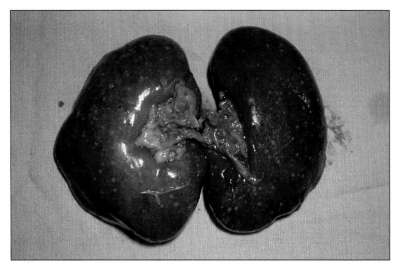

FIGURE 2-41 Gross specimen of kidney in acute severe complicated pyelonephritis, showing multiple microabscesses. The surface of the kidney is dotted with widespread, small, yellowish microabscesses. In adults, complicated pyelonephritis occurs in both men and women, often the elderly. It is generally the result of structural or functional abnormalities (prostatitis in men, obstruction, calculi, neurologic diseases, vesicoureteral reflux, impaired renal function), urologic manipulations (drainage devices, urinary catheters, urinary instrumentation, renal transplantation), underlying diseases (diabetes, immunosuppression or immunodeficiencies, sickle cell traits, or cystic renal diseases). In contrast, patients with uncomplicated pyelonephritis do not have these underlying predisposing factors. In patients with uncomplicated pyelonephritis, bacterial virulence factors play a more significant role.

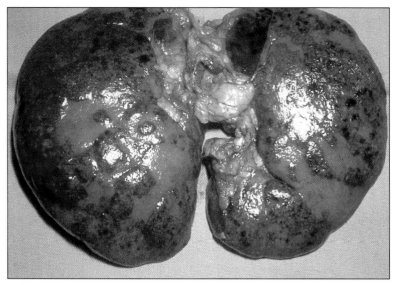

FIGURE 2-42 Gross view of kidneys in disseminated intravascular coagulation. Disseminated intravascular coagulation, whether associated with severe pyelonephritis or other infectious diseases, may precipitate renal failure and induce severe renal lesions. Note the multiple hemorrhagic spots on the surface of the kidneys, associated with diffuse microthrombi within the parenchyma.

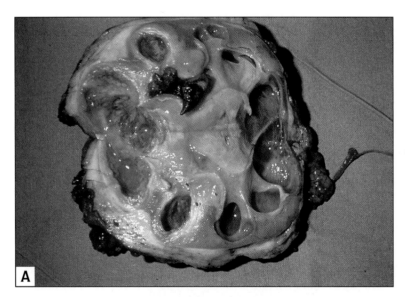

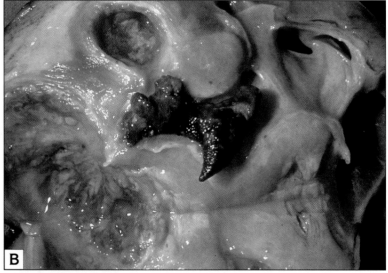

FIGURE 2-43 Gross specimen of kidney demonstrating xanthogranulomatous pyelonephritis. **A** and **B**, The kidney also shows multiple abscesses, dilatation of the calyceal system, and necrosis and scarring of the renal tissue associated with a staghorn calculus.

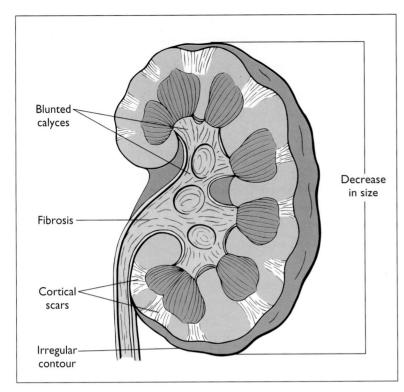

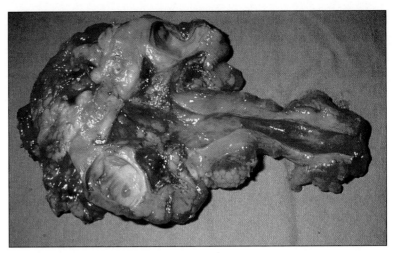

FIGURE 2-45 Gross specimen of kidney in chronic pyelonephritis, showing severe scarring atrophy, dilation of the pyelocalyceal cavities, fibrous thickening of the ureteral wall, and hyperemia of the mucosa.

FIGURE 2-44 Diagram of the histopathologic changes in the kidney observed in chronic pyelonephritis.

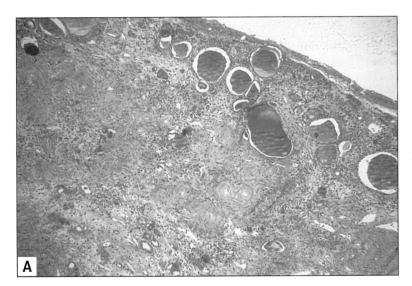

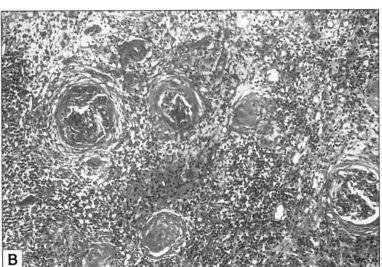

FIGURE 2-46 Histopathologic examination in chronic pyelonephritis. **A,** Kidney section shows massive fibrous scarring throughout the parenchyma with tubular atrophy and dilatation (thyroidization), glomerular sclerosis, arteriosclerosis, and chronic interstitial inflammation. **B,** Higher magnification of the kidney section shows severe infiltration of lymphocytes and plasma cells; glomerular, periglomerular, and interstitial fibrosis with extensive tubule loss; and atrophy.

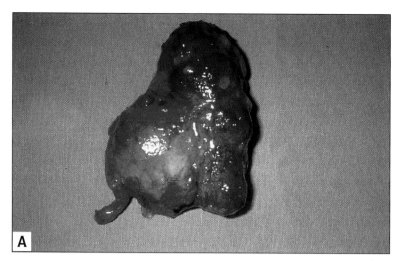
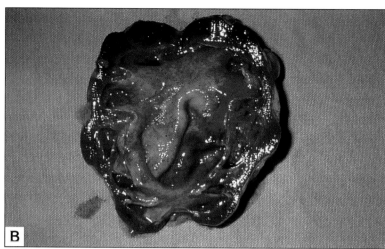

FIGURE 2-47 Gross specimen of kidney showing chronic pyelonephritis with hydronephrosis. **A** and **B**, There is swelling of the pyelocalyceal region, dilatation of the kidney, blunting of the papillae, and atrophy of the cortex with an irregular scarred surface.

Renal function abnormalities associated with pyelonephritis

Inability to concentrate urine (transient)
Renal insufficiency (rare)

FIGURE 2-48 Renal function abnormalities associated with pyelonephritis. Very few changes in renal function are associated with pyelonephritis. Most people with severe acute pyelonephritis demonstrate a limited capacity of the kidney to concentrate urine, but this abnormality can usually be corrected with appropriate antibiotic therapy. An increased production of prostaglandins associated with the inflammatory process may explain these abnormalities. Although renal failure may be the result of severe obstruction or "severe chronic" pyelonephritis, it is almost never a complication of acute uncomplicated pyelonephritis.

TREATMENT

Uropathogens and their susceptibility to antibiotics used in pyelonephritis

	Escherichia coli (492)*, %	*Klebsiella pneumoniae* (105), %	*Proteus mirabilis* (37), %	*Pseudomonas aeruginosa* (78), %	*Serratia marcescens* (40), %
Aminoglycosides					
Gentamicin	98	99	100	96	100
β-Lactams					
Ampicillin	67	4	84	0	2
Ceftriaxone	100	100	100	72	95
Aztreonam	99	100	100	94	95
Ticarcillin/clavulanate	98	100	100	95	97
Imipenem/cilastatin	100	100	100	91	100
Fluoroquinolones					
Ciprofloxacin	100	100	100	100	100
Other antibiotics					
Trimethoprim-sulfamethoxazole	91	96	92	3	98

*Number of isolates. All these bacteria were isolated in the blood of patients.

FIGURE 2-49 Uropathogens and their susceptibility to antibiotics used in pyelonephritis. The susceptibility of *Escherichia coli* to antibiotics is changing. *E. coli* resistance to ampicillin, amoxicillin, and first-generation cephalosporins is increasing rapidly (25%–35%) so that these drugs cannot be considered anymore as the first choice for empirical treatment of pyelonephritis. In North America, *E. coli* and many other Enterobacteriaceae are still susceptible to trimethoprim-sulfamethoxazole (TMP-SMX), but resistance is rising (10%–15%). In many parts of Europe, *E. coli* is highly resistant to TMP-SMX. Although variable from country to country, aminoglycosides and the quinolones are still, in general, highly effective against many gram-negative bacteria responsible for uncomplicated and complicated pyelonephritis. (*Adapted from* Chamberland *et al.* [7].)

Susceptibility of gram-positive coccal pyelonephritis

Enterococci
  Increasing resistance to ampicillin, vancomycin,
      aminoglycosides
Staphylococcus aureus
  Rare urinary pathogen
  Mostly methicillin-susceptible
Staphylococcus epidermidis
  Usually catheter-related
  Frequently methicillin-resistant

FIGURE 2-50 Susceptibility of gram-positive coccal pyelonephritis. Enterococci, *Staphylococcus aureus*, *S. epidermidis*, and even *Corynebacterium* group D2 are now responsible for an increasing percentage of uncomplicated and complicated pyelonephritis, and these gram-positive bacteria may be highly resistant to antibiotics. The enterococci are becoming more resistant to ampicillin and aminoglycosides, but both agents are still first-line therapies until susceptibility data are available. Although vancomycin and teicoplanin may neutralize the enterococci, there are almost no data on their efficacy in pyelonephritis, although vancomycin penetrates the renal parenchyma well. Imipenem-cilastatin may also be used. A high percentage of *S. epidermidis* and an increasing number of *S. aureus* are now resistant to methicillin. Vancomycin or teicoplanin are the appropriate alternatives. For some vancomycin-resistant enterococci, RP 59500 (Synercid), a new experimental streptogramin, may become a proper choice in the near future.

Intrarenal pharmacology of antibiotics used in pyelonephritis

Antibiotics	Doses, *mg/kg*	Maximal renal levels, *µg/g of tissue*	Ratio renal/serum	Persistence in kidney
Aminoglycosides				
Gentamicin	10	40/630	3/70	Up to 1 yr (365 days)
Netilmicin	10	240/720	16/70	> 25 days
Tobramycin	40	250	30–40	> 10 days
β-Lactams				
Ampicillin	100	65	1	< 4 hrs
Ceftriaxone	100	72	0.65	< 6 hrs
Quinolones				
Norfloxacin	400 mg	16	3.8	No data
Enoxacin	400 mg	16.1	7.7	No data
Fleroxacin	50	45/60	3/5	> 24 hrs
Temafloxacin	25	60	2	< 12 hrs
Other antibiotics				
Trimethoprim	10	32	20	< 16 hrs
Sulfamethoxazole	50	50	0.4	< 24 hrs
Vancomycin	20	85	2	> 24 hrs
Daptomycin	10	4	0.2	< 12 hrs

FIGURE 2-51 Intrarenal pharmacology of antibiotics used in pyelonephritis. Whether a drug must reach inhibitory concentrations in the bloodstream as well as in urine and renal tissue to be effective in the treatment of pyelonephritis is still debatable. Early investigations have shown that low doses of oral antimicrobial agents, including penicillins, nitrofurantoin, and tetracyclines, were effective in the therapy for pyelonephritis as long as urinary levels remained above the minimum inhibitory concentration of the antibiotic against the pathogens, even though serum levels were insufficient to inhibit the pathogens. Little information is available on the intrarenal distribution of antibiotics in humans. Most of our knowledge on the intrarenal pharmacokinetics of drugs is derived from animal experiments. As shown in this figure, noticeable differences exist in the disposition and persistence of various antibiotics in the kidney parenchyma. Both serum and urine concentrations are poor predictors of the levels of antimicrobial agents in the cortex, medulla, and papilla. Furthermore, the mere presence of infection and endotoxin may modify the intrarenal pharmacokinetics of antimicrobial agents. (*Adapted from* Bergeron [3].)

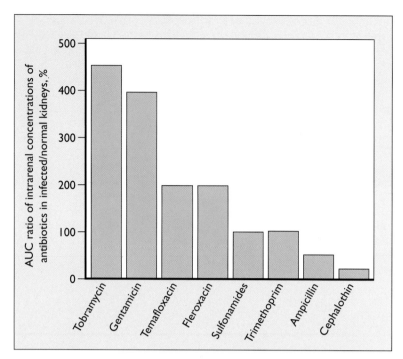

FIGURE 2-52 Pyelonephritis effects on antibiotic pharmacokinetics. In choosing an antimicrobial therapy for pyelonephritis, one has to consider that renal infection modifies the intrarenal pharmacokinetics of antibiotics. β-Lactams such as cephalosporins and penicillins are affected negatively and are recovered in less concentration in the infected kidney compared with noninfected renal tissue. (Ratio in percentage of area under the concentrations curve [AUC] of different antibiotics within infected kidney and the AUC of these antibiotics in noninfected kidneys is < 100%.) Trimethoprim-sulfamethoxazole is not affected by infection, whereas quinolones and aminoglycosides are recovered in higher concentration in infected tissue, most likely explaining, at least in part, their good efficacy in pyelonephritis.

Aminoglycosides: Implications of renal pharmacokinetics

High renal medulla levels contribute to superior therapeutics in resistant pyelonephritis

Persistent high medulla levels exert continued pharmacologic synergy with β-lactams, even after only 3 days of aminoglycoside therapy

FIGURE 2-53 Aminoglycosides: Implications of renal pharmacokinetics. The unique pharmacology of aminoglycosides provides for high drug concentrations in the kidney, which persist long after cessation of therapy, and for a reduced risk of toxicity [8]. To take advantage of the pharmacologic benefits, we reduced therapy with aminoglycosides to 3 days and continued on with ampicillin alone. Treatment with 3 days on aminoglycoside, in combination with ampicillin for 14 days, gave similar results to 14 days of gentamicin, suggesting not only antibacterial synergism but pharmacologic synergism. In our studies, the new quinolone fleroxacin was as effective as aminoglycoside therapy. Although aminoglycosides are commonly used in therapy for severe urinary tract infections in humans, there are very limited data comparing the efficacy of a few days of aminoglycosides (associated or not with another antibiotic) and a quinolone given intravenously followed by an oral agent for a total of 2 weeks. This sequential therapy allows for early discharge and is cost effective.

Comparative sequential therapy (intravenous followed by oral) in 41 patients with pyelonephritis

| | Enoxacin* | | Tobramycin-ampicillin† | |
	Clinical efficacy, *n(%)*	Bacteriologic efficacy, *n(%)*	Clinical efficacy, *n(%)*	Bacteriologic efficacy, *n(%)*
No. of patients	23	22	18	18
Cure	19 (83)	16 (73)	16 (89)	14 (76)
Failure	4 (17)	6 (27)	2 (11)	4 (24)

*Enoxacin intravenously (IV) for 3 days (300–500 mg IV every 12 hrs) followed by oral enoxacin (400 mg twice a day for 10 days).

†Tobramycin IV for 3 days (1.5 mg/kg IV every 8 hrs) plus ampicillin (1 g IV every 6 hrs) followed by oral amoxicillin (500 mg every 8 hrs) or trimethoprim-sulfamethoxazole (160/800 mg twice a day for 10 days).

FIGURE 2-54 Comparative sequential therapy in 41 patients with pyelonephritis. In a comparative randomized study, we have recently shown that ± 3 days of tobramycin associated with either ampicillin or trimethoprim-sulfamethoxozole (TMP-SMX), followed by oral therapy with either amoxicillin or TMP-SMX based on susceptibility pattern of the bacteria, gave identical outcome to intravenous enoxacin followed by oral enoxacin. More than 80% of patients were clinically cured of their severe pyelonephritis with both regimens. Based on these human and animal experiments, many believe that to cure pyelonephritis, it is necessary to reach inhibitory levels both in the kidneys and urine of such patients. Moreover, if septicemia is present, drugs must be inhibitory in serum as well. Severe pyelonephritis necessitates hospitalization. Three days of parenteral aminoglycosides, alone or in combination with intravenous ampicillin or TMP-SMX, followed by oral therapy with these agents is probably equivalent to 3 days of an intravenous quinolone followed by a quinolone orally. Aminoglycosides can also be given as a single daily dose. (*Adapted from* Bergeron [3].)

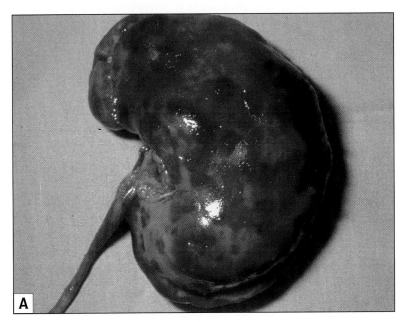

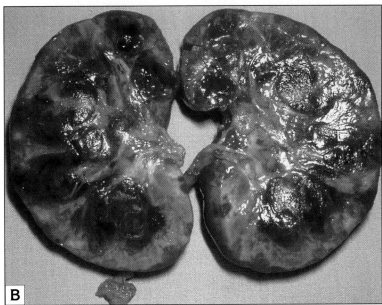

FIGURE 2-67 Pyelonephritis in renal transplantation. **A** and **B**, Urinary infections occur in 30% to 50% of transplant recipients, often within 2 months of surgery, and recurrences are frequent. Immunosuppression and vesicourethral reflux resulting from urologic manipulation are the triggering factors of these infections. A high level of suspicion is needed, because these patients often have silent pyelonephritis. There are very limited data on the management of these patients. Either trimethoprim-sulfamethoxazole (TMP-SMX) or a quinolone would be given, the latter if a nosocomial pathogen is suspected or identified. In severe cases, one should start with intravenous therapy using either an aminoglycoside or a quinolone followed by oral antibiotics. Prophylaxis with either TMP-SMX or a quinolone has been shown effective to prevent urinary tract infections in this population. Pyelonephritis may be associated with acute rejection of the graft.

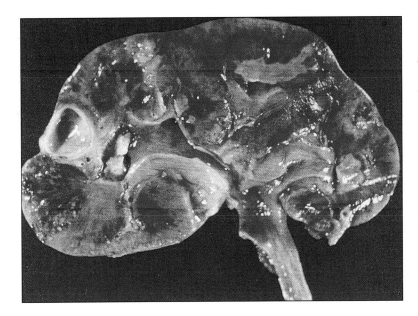

FIGURE 2-68 Acute necrotizing papillitis in a patient with diabetes. Marked inflammation and edematous papilla and calyces and multiple abscesses are observed within the cortex and medulla. In the era before antimicrobial agents, postmortem studies documented that the occurrence of pyelonephritis in diabetes was five times that in nondiabetic patients. Once infected, diabetic patients may develop very severe diseases. Urinary stones, glycosuria, limited vascularity of the renal medulla, and impaired phagocytosis increase the susceptibility of these patients to pyelonephritis. Pyelonephritis is also a common cause of coma, ketoacidosis, and hyperosmolality. In patients with diabetes, asymptomatic bacteriuria may precede pyelonephritis. Papillary necrosis and severe septicemia frequently complicate pyelonephritis in this population. More intensive and prolonged therapy with bactericidal agents is required with aminoglycosides, quinolones, trimethoprim-sulfamethaxozole, or newer β-lactams. Emphysematous pyelonephritis in diabetic patients is associated with a high mortality. It can be recognized on flat-plate films of the abdomen and may necessitate life-saving nephrectomy.

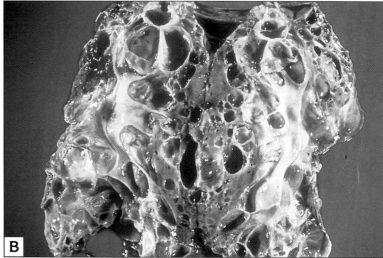

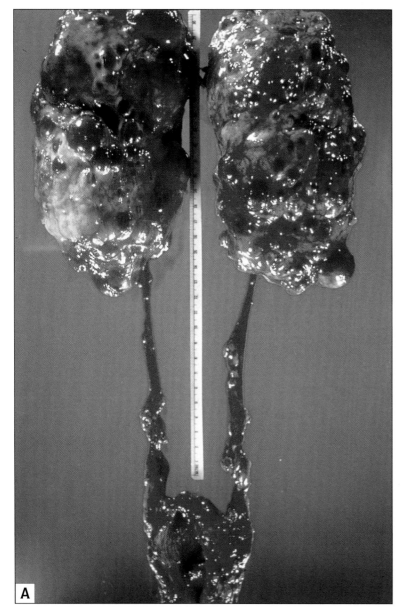

FIGURE 2-69 Pyelonephritis in cystic renal disease. **A** and **B,** Poly-cystic kidneys may get infected and form abscesses. These multiple cysts become a closed environment with limited vascular supply that predispose to infection and abscess formation. Imaging studies (computed tomography and ultrasound) can distinguish between a complicated and a noncomplicated cyst but cannot differentiate between a hemorrhagic and an infectious cyst. Long-term follow-up of patients with cystic renal disease has shown that more than half of these patients will develop bacteriuria. Pyelonephritis with intrarenal or perirenal abscesses are common. The response to therapy is generally poor, because these infections are in a closed environment where diffusion of antibiotics is limited and host response poor. Trimethoprim-sulfamethaxozole or a quinolone would seem appropriate. Therapy should be given for 6 weeks.

High failure rate for therapy in pyelonephritis

Very high, approximately one third at 3 mos
Causes (relapse or reinfection)
  Indwelling catheters
  Failure to relieve/remove obstruction, calculi, stasis, reflux, etc.
  Underlying structural anomaly (*eg,* cysts)
  Resistant organisms (rare)
  Failure to provide sufficiently prolonged antibacterial therapy

FIGURE 2-70 High failure rate for therapy in pyelonephritis. The failure rate in the treatment of pyelonephritis is extremely high, with most failures occurring in complicated pyelonephritis. In the absence of obstruction or foreign bodies, failure of therapy has been attributed to bacterial resistance, presence of L-forms, reinfection with a new pathogen, or the use of appropriate antibiotics for an insufficient duration. Bacterial antibiotic resistance is rarely the cause of therapy failure in pyelonephritis. Close follow-up is required.

ACKNOWLEDGMENTS

The authors thank Dr. Nicole Plamondon (radiologist, Hôtel-Dieu de Québec), Dr. Louise Côté, Dr. Michel Tremblay, Gisèle Chassé, Marthe Bernier, Odette Guibord, and Lise Villeneuve (Centre Hospitalier de L'Université Laval) for their contributions.

REFERENCES

1. Eroschenko VP: *Atlas of Histology with Functional Correlations*, 7th ed. Philadelphia: Lea & Febiger; 1993:229.

2. Tardif M, Beauchamp D, Bergeron Y, *et al.*: L-651,391, a potent leukotriene inhibitor, controls inflammatory process in *E. coli* pyelonephritis. *Antimicrob Agents Chemother* 1994, 38:1555–1560.

3. Bergeron MG: Treatment of pyelonephritis. *Med Clin North Am* 1995, 79:619–649.

4. Huang JJ, Sung JM, Chen KW, *et al.*: Acute bacterial nephritis: A clinicoradiologic correlation based on computed tomography. *Am J Med* 1992, 93:289–298.

5. Johnson HR, Vincent LM, Wang K, *et al.*: Renal ultrasonographic correlates of acute pyelonephritis. *Clin Infect Dis* 1992, 14:15–22.

6. Huang JJ, Sung JM, Kuan-Wen C, *et al.*: Acute bacterial nephritis: A clinico-radiologic correlation based on computed tomography. *Am J Med* 1992, 93:289–298.

7. Chamberland S, L'Écuyer J, Lessard C, *et al.*: Antibiotic susceptibility profiles of 941 gram-negative bacteria isolated from septicemia patients throughout Canada. *Clin Infect Dis* 1992, 15:615–628.

8. Bergeron MG, Marois Y: Benefit from high levels of gentamicin in the treatment of *E. coli* pyelonephritis. *Kidney Int* 1986, 30:481.

SELECTED BIBLIOGRAPHY

Bailey RR: Duration of antimicrobial treatment and the use of drug combinations for the treatment of uncomplicated acute pyelonephritis. *Infection* 1994, 22(suppl 1):S50.

Bergeron MG: Treatment of pyelonephritis in adults. *Med Clin North Am* 1995, 79:619–649.

Lipsky BA: Urinary tract infections in men: Epidemiology, pathophysiology, diagnosis, and treatment. *Ann Intern Med* 1989, 110:138.

Sobel JD, Kaye D: Urinary tract infection. *In* Mandell GL, Bennett JE, Dolin R (eds.): *Principles and Practice of Infectious Diseases*, 4th ed. New York: Churchill Livingstone; 1995:662.

Stamm WE, Hooton TM: Management of urinary tract infections in adults. *N Engl J Med* 1993, 329:1328.

CHAPTER 3

Complicated Urinary Tract Infections

Lindsay E. Nicolle

A. Complicated urinary tract infection: Definition

Urinary tract infection occurring in persons with functional or anatomic abnormalities of the urinary tract or with catheterization

B. Complicated urinary tract infection: Clinical situations

Presence of an indwelling catheter or use of intermittent catheterization
> 100 mL of residual urine retained after voiding
Obstructive uropathy due to bladder outlet obstruction, calculus, or other causes
Vesicle ureteral reflux or other urologic abnormalities, including surgically created ileal loops
Azotemia due to intrinsic renal disease
Renal transplantation

FIGURE 3-1 Definition of complicated urinary tract infections. **A**, A complicated urinary tract infection is defined as one that occurs in a person with a preexisting functional or anatomic abnormality of the urinary tract or with catheterization. **B**, Specific clinical situations defining a complicated urinary tract infection [1].

Microbiologic diagnosis of complicated urinary tract infection

Symptomatic
$\geq 10^5$ cfu/mL organisms
Lower quantitative counts
Diuresis
Renal failure
Selected organisms
Asymptomatic
$\geq 10^5$ cfu/mL in two consecutive specimens

cfu—colony-forming units.

FIGURE 3-2 Microbiologic diagnosis of complicated urinary tract infection. In patients with symptoms of urinary tract infection or with fever and flank pain, the isolation of $\geq 10^5$ colony-forming units (cfu) of organisms per mL of urine is diagnostic of urinary tract infection. On occasion, lower quantitative counts occur in subjects with symptomatic infection. These may include subjects with diuresis, renal failure, or infection with selected organisms, such as *Candida albicans* or *Staphylococcus saprophyticus*. For the diagnosis of asymptomatic bacteriuria, two consecutive urine specimens with $\geq 10^5$ cfu/mL of one or more organisms is necessary [1].

Microbiology of complicated urinary tract infection

Pathogen	Louie *et al.* [2]	Cox [3]
Escherichia coli	80	49
Klebsiella spp	14	29
Citrobacter spp	9	12
Enterobacter spp	8	20
Proteus mirabilis	10	12
Pseudomonas aeruginosa	3	10
Other gram-negative organisms	9	9
Staphylococcus aureus	3	—
Coagulase-negative staphylococci	2	—
Enterococcus spp	9	1

FIGURE 3-3 Microbiology of complicated urinary tract infection. Organisms isolated from subjects in two studies of complicated urinary tract infection are summarized [2,3].

Microbiologic aspects of complicated urinary tract infection

Non–*Escherichia coli* infections common
Increased likelihood of resistant organisms
Increased likelihood of polymicrobial infection

FIGURE 3-4 Microbiologic aspects of complicated urinary tract infection. The microbiology of complicated urinary tract infections varies from that of uncomplicated urinary tract infections. Although *Escherichia coli* remains an important pathogen, the microbiology is generally characterized by an increased variety of organisms and organisms of increasing antimicrobial resistance. In addition, organisms frequently lack typical virulence factors required for establishing themselves in the normal urinary tract. Distribution of organisms and antimicrobial susceptibilities may vary with different institutions. Isolation of more than one organism occurs frequently in patients with complicated urinary infection.

Principles of antimicrobial management of complicated urinary tract infection

Therapy guided by culture
Antimicrobial agents with urinary excretion should be used
Short-term therapy not appropriate
High recurrence rate
Prolonged therapy may be required
  Prophylaxis: prevent reinfection
  Suppression: prevent symptomatic episode or stone enlargement

FIGURE 3-5 Principles of antimicrobial management of complicated urinary tract infection. Because of the variety of organisms and increased likelihood of antimicrobial resistance in complicated urinary tract infections, urine culture and susceptibility testing to direct antimicrobial selection are essential. Agents documented to be effective in clinical trials should be used, with an initial duration of therapy of 7 to 14 days. The expected recurrence rate at 4 to 6 weeks is 40% to 50%. Prolonged therapy is necessary in some patients to prevent reinfection (prophylaxis) or symptomatic recurrences in subjects in whom infection cannot be eradicated (suppression).

OBSTRUCTION

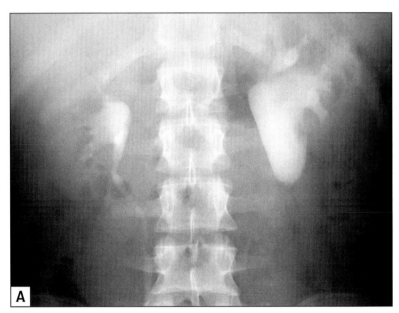 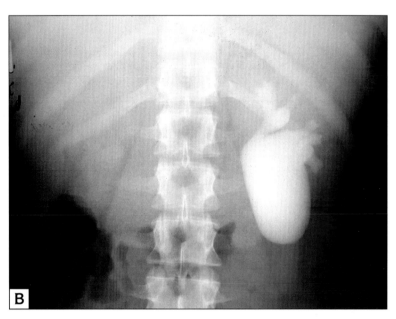

FIGURE 3-6 Pelviureteric junction obstruction demonstrated by intravenous pyelography. Obstruction to urine flow at any level in the urinary tract promotes urinary tract infection. **A**, On the 15-minute intravenous pyelogram film, contrast is excreted well in the right kidney, but the left kidney has a dilated pelvis and calyceal system. **B**, At the 4-hour intravenous pyelogram film, there is no further contrast remaining in the right kidney, but the left kidney retains contrast in the pelvis and calyceal system. The obstruction is at the level of the pelviureteric junction.

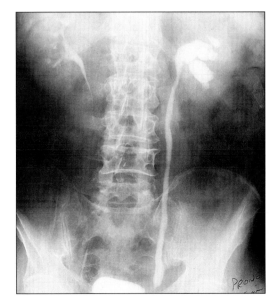

FIGURE 3-7 Intravenous pyelogram showing ureteric stricture due to renal tuberculosis. Ureteric strictures may be associated with proximal dilatation of the urinary system and urinary tract infection because of incomplete emptying. This prone 45-minute intravenous pyelogram film demonstrates amputation of the infundibula to the left upper pole and a stricture of the distal left ureter. In this case, the ureteric stricture is due to tuberculosis of the genitourinary tract.

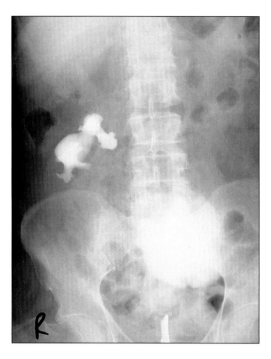

FIGURE 3-8 Intravenous pyelogram film showing hydronephrosis from extrinsic obstruction. Obstruction occurring within the genitourinary tract may be either intrinsic (*ie*, within the hollow structures of the renal pelvis, ureters, bladder, or urethra) or extrinsic. Tumors or other masses in the pelvis may obstruct the ureters. This intravenous pyelogram shows mild hydronephrosis of the right kidney and a severely hydronephrotic pelvic kidney in a patient with radiation fibrosis following radiation therapy for prostatic carcinoma.

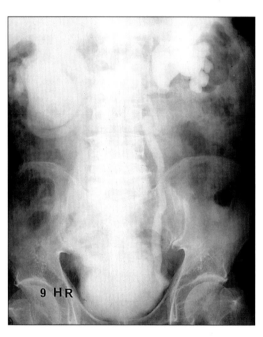

FIGURE 3-9 Prostatic obstruction, seen on intravenous pyelogram film. In elderly men, prostatic hypertrophy with obstruction is a common cause of impaired voiding and recurrent urinary tract infection. In this intravenous pyelogram, a man aged 92 years shows gross enlargement of the bladder and dilatation of the collecting system of the kidneys and ureters secondary to prostatic obstruction. The degree of dilatation suggests obstruction is long standing.

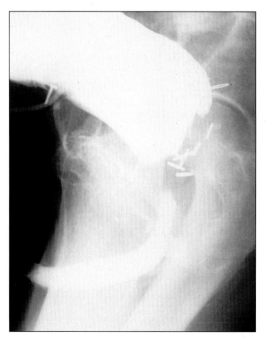

FIGURE 3-10 Urethral stricture seen on cystourethrogram. Urethral strictures are another cause of genitourinary obstruction. In this cystourethrogram, a severe stricture approximately 2 cm in length of the urethra is demonstrated. This patient developed the stricture following transurethral resection of the prostate for prostatic carcinoma. Although urinary tract infection may occur due to obstruction to voiding from stricture, symptoms associated with the stricture itself, including hesitancy, frequency, and occasionally dysuria, may be similar to symptoms of urinary tract infection.

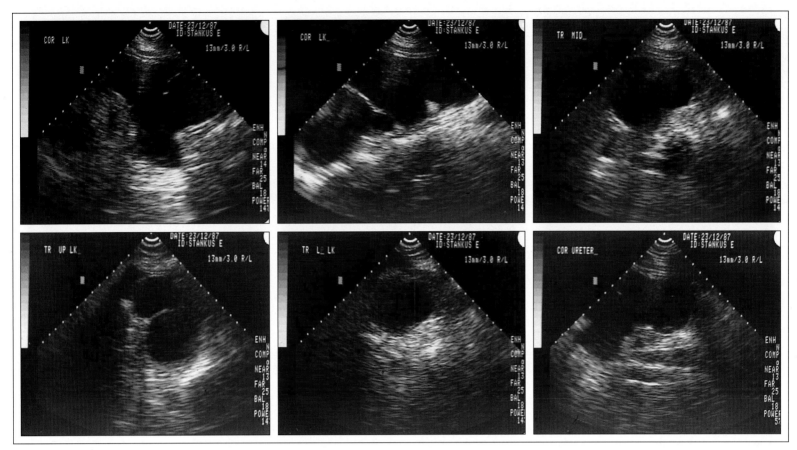

FIGURE 3-11 Renal ultrasound showing hydronephrosis secondary to obstruction. Hydronephrosis secondary to obstruction may be acute or chronic. The lack of free urinary drainage may promote urinary tract infection and complicate efforts to treat such infection. This ultrasound shows gross hydronephrosis of the left kidney, with a markedly dilated left ureter and loss of renal parenchyma. An intravenous pyelogram of the same patient showed a nonfunctioning left kidney, and retrograde pyelogram showed only a small amount of contrast visualized in the distal 1 cm of the left ureter. The obstruction was likely of 10 years' duration and secondary to ligation of the left ureter at a previous hysterectomy.

CALCULI

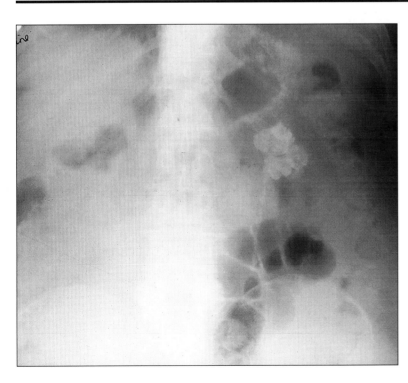

FIGURE 3-12 Staghorn calculus seen on abdominal radiograph. Staghorn calculi are "infection stones" (struvite and calcium carbonate apatite), produced in association with infection with urease-producing organisms, primarily *Proteus mirabilis*. These are generally large calculi that follow the contours of the renal pelvis and may destroy the kidney. This abdominal film shows a staghorn calculus of the left kidney with associated calcification of the left upper ureter in a woman presenting with recurrent abdominal pain.

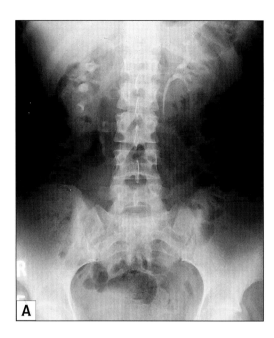
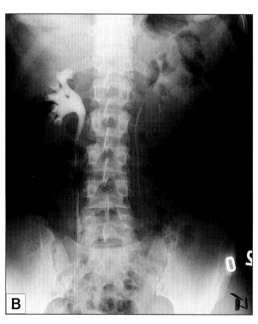

FIGURE 3-13 Intravenous pyelograms showing ureteric stone with pyelonephritis. Renal stones are usually passed in the ureter and may cause ureteric obstruction. Occasionally, this obstruction will be complicated by infection. These intravenous pyelogram films were obtained from a woman aged 18 years presenting with right flank pain and fever. **A,** On the 5-minute film, there is a calcified density overlying the right transverse process of L3, which is a stone in the right ureter. **B,** On the 20-minute film, delayed excretion of contrast with some dilatation of the upper renal collecting system is seen with an irregularity of the ureter at the level of the stone.

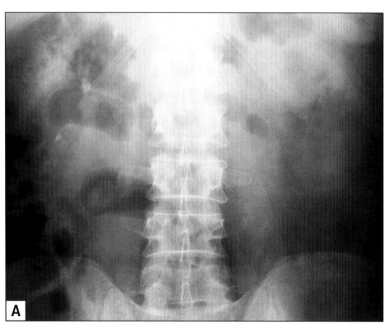
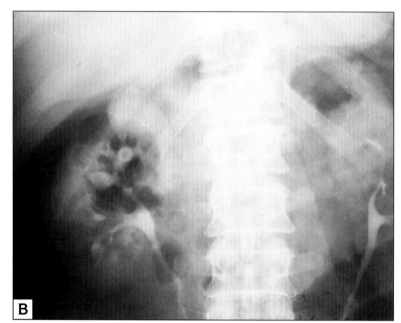

FIGURE 3-14 Renal stones causing localized calyceal obstruction. Stones within the renal pelvis may cause local renal obstruction. **A,** This plain film of the abdomen reveals two calcified lesions in the area of the right kidney. **B,** A 5-minute intravenous pyelo-gram film shows evidence of obstruction of the upper pole of the right kidney due to one of the renal stones. The other stone lies free in the lower right renal pelvis.

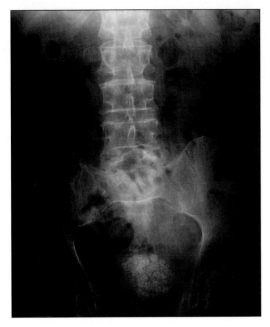

FIGURE 3-15 Bladder stones seen on plain abdominal radiograph. Bladder calculi usually occur in individuals with chronic urinary tract infection with urease-producing organisms. They occur frequently in individuals with chronic indwelling urethral catheters and were previously an important problem in patients with spinal cord injury. This plain film of the abdomen from a paraplegic man displays multiple calculi in the bladder. Removal of these stones is necessary if urinary tract infection is to be successfully treated in these patients.

NEUROGENIC BLADDER

UTI in spinal cord injury with neurogenic bladder

Patients
  64 catheter-free subjects
  Monthly urine cultures
  18 with intermittent catheter, 46 with condom
Prevalence: 57.4%
Overall incidence: 18.4 UTI/person-year
Febrile infection: 1.82 episodes/person-year

UTI—urinary tract infection.

FIGURE 3-16 Urinary tract infection (UTI) in spinal cord injury. Subjects with neurogenic bladder are at high risk for UTIs. To prevent reflux and renal damage, a low-pressure bladder with intermittent complete voiding must be maintained. This state may be achieved by intermittent catheterization or by surgical procedures such as sphincterotomy. In a few cases, long-term indwelling catheters may be required. One large group of individuals with neurogenic bladder are those with spinal cord injuries. Many of these patients are now managed with intermittent catheterization, although, with men, condom drainage with or without sphincterotomy is a possibility. Despite low pressures and low residua in the bladder, UTI still occurs with high frequency in these groups, although it is less frequently associated with renal damage. In a study by Waites and colleagues [4], 64 spinal cord-injured patients with neurogenic bladders, 18 maintained on intermittent catheterization and 46 with condom catheter drainage, were followed with monthly urine cultures for up to 1 year. The overall prevalence of UTIs in all urine cultures was 57.4%. In addition, there were 18.4 episodes of UTI per person-year, although only 1.82 episodes per person-year were febrile infection.

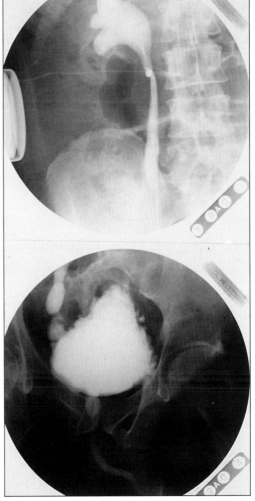

FIGURE 3-17 Voiding cystourethrogram showing reflux in a patient with spinal cord injury. This voiding cysto-urethrogram is from a man aged 44 years with a 4-year history of spinal cord injury. The *bottom panel* shows the characteristic observations in a high-pressure uninhibited neurogenic bladder with trabeculations and diverticuli, with reflux of contrast up the right ureter. The *top panel* shows reflux extending up to the right calyceal system. The right ureter shows dilatation with blunting of calyces due to the reflux.

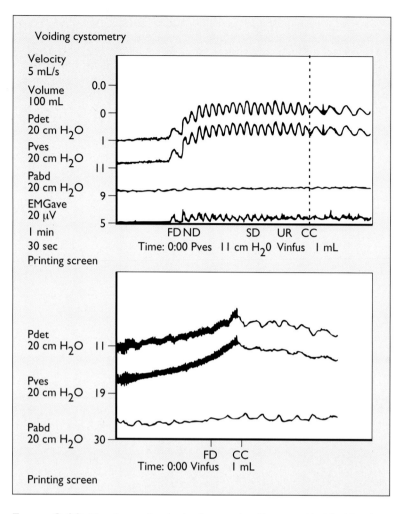

Voiding cystometry

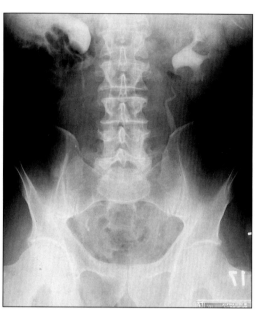

FIGURE 3-18 Urodynamic study demonstrating spastic bladder in spinal cord injury. A neurogenic bladder may be associated with

uninhibited detrusor contractions at relatively low volumes. Voiding cystometrograms in two spinal cord-injured patients demonstrate high-pressure uninhibited bladders. The *top panel* shows a patient with continuous detrusor activity with any volume in the bladder; the *bottom panel* shows larger uninhibited contractions occurring after an initial period with no detrusor activity. (CC—maximum cystometric capacity; EMGave—average electromyogram; FD—first desire to void; ND—normal desire to void; Pabd—pressure abdomen; Pdet—pressure detrusor; Pves—pressure vesicle; SD—strong desire to void; UR—urgency, vinfus—velocity of infusion.)

FIGURE 3-19 Neurogenic bladder in multiple sclerosis. Patients with neurogenic bladders may also have flaccid, areflexic bladders. Subjects with flaccid bladders may have very large volumes and are subject to recurrent infection. This 17-minute intravenous pyelogram film demonstrates a huge soft-tissue mass in the central abdomen that is a distended bladder in a patient with neurogenic bladder due to multiple sclerosis.

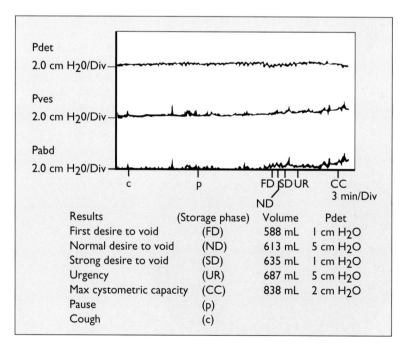

Results	(Storage phase)	Volume	Pdet
First desire to void	(FD)	588 mL	1 cm H_2O
Normal desire to void	(ND)	613 mL	5 cm H_2O
Strong desire to void	(SD)	635 mL	1 cm H_2O
Urgency	(UR)	687 mL	5 cm H_2O
Max cystometric capacity	(CC)	838 mL	2 cm H_2O
Pause	(p)		
Cough	(c)		

FIGURE 3-20 Urodynamic study showing decreased detrusor activity (flaccid bladder). A flaccid neurogenic bladder is associated with large bladder volumes and limited detrusor activity. This urodynamic study is one example of such a flaccid bladder. The detrusor pressure (Pdet) is only 2 cm H_2O despite a total volume of > 800 mL infused into the bladder. When this patient was catheterized prior to the urodynamic study being done, the volume in the bladder was 950 mL. (Div—division; Pabd—pressure abdomen; Pves—pressure vesicle.)

DIABETES MELLITUS

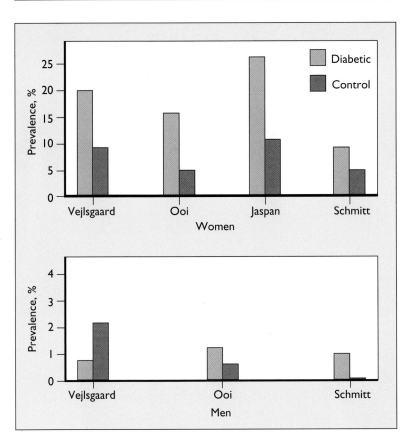

FIGURE 3-21 Prevalence of asymptomatic bacteriuria in patients with diabetes. Several studies enrolling relatively large numbers of subjects and reporting on the prevalence of bacteriuria in diabetic compared with control populations are summarized in this figure. For women, studies generally report a prevalence of bacteriuria two to three times higher in diabetics than in controls. This is not the case for diabetic men. In addition, as for most populations, the prevalence of bacteriuria in women is substantially higher than men. The clinical significance of this increased prevalance of bacteriuria in diabetic women is not clear [5–8].

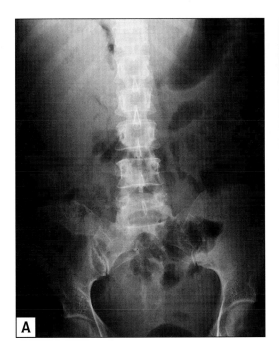 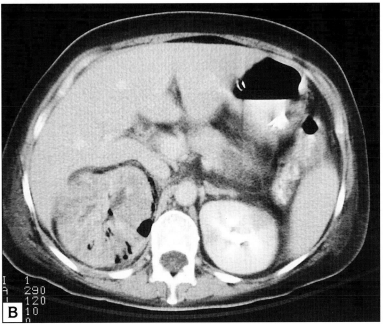

FIGURE 3-22 Emphysematous pyelonephritis in a patient with diabetes. A rare presentation of urinary tract infection in diabetic patients is that of emphysematous pyelonephritis. This condition occurs in the presence of hyperglycemia with glucose excreted in the urine. Uropathogens may produce gas in the presence of elevated glucose. **A,** In this plain film of the abdomen, an elderly diabetic woman has evidence of gas surrounding, and in the parenchyma of, the right kidney. **B,** The computed tomography scan shows an enlarged, inflamed, right kidney with air within the parenchyma and subcapsular space.

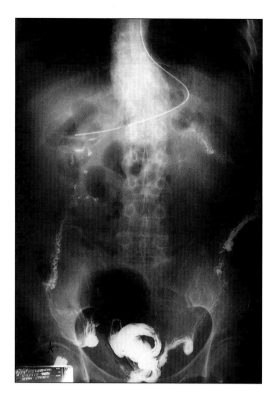

FIGURE 3-23 Abdominal radiograph showing emphysematous cystitis in a patient with diabetes. Emphysematous cystitis is an infection of the bladder with production of air by the infecting organisms. It occurs in diabetics with hyperglycemia. In the presence of the increased sugar in the urine, gram-negative organisms may produce gas. This plain abdominal film shows barium in the colon from a previous barium examination. There also is a large air-containing mass in the pelvis, which is the bladder. The patient was a diabetic woman aged 61 years with a *Klebsiella pneumoniae* infection.

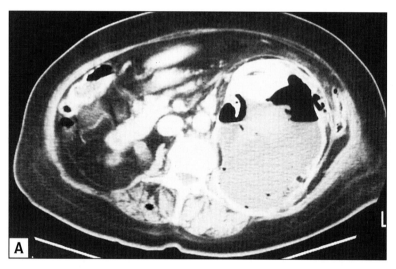

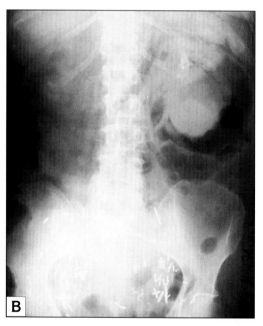

FIGURE 3-24 Perinephric abscess in a woman with diabetes. Perinephric abscesses occur in the space between the kidney and Gerota's fascia. They may occur following hematogenous spread through bloodstream infections or secondary to obstruction of the urinary tract and renal infection. **A,** A plain film of the abdomen of a diabetic woman aged 76 years with a prior history of bladder carcinoma. She presented with a 4-month history of illness and passed a bladder stone 4 days before presentation. The abdominal kidney, ureter, and bladder film reveals a large left-upper-quadrant mass with air present within it. **B,** The computed tomography scan demonstrates the huge mass replacing the left kidney with air-fluid levels within it.

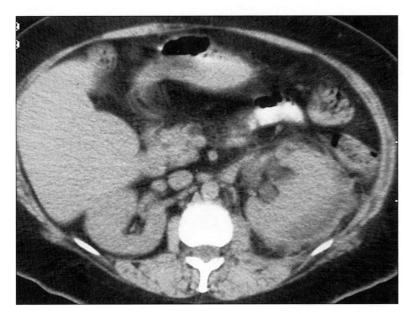

FIGURE 3-25 Computed tomography scan showing a left perinephric abscess. This elderly diabetic woman presented with a 1-year history of chronic urinary tract infection associated initially with a left renal pelvis stone and, subsequently, a left ureteric stricture requiring repeated manipulations. On this occasion, the patient presented with sepsis. The computed tomography scan reveals a moderate left-sided hydronephrosis with a large subcapsular and perinephric abscess of the left kidney.

CONGENITAL ABNORMALITIES

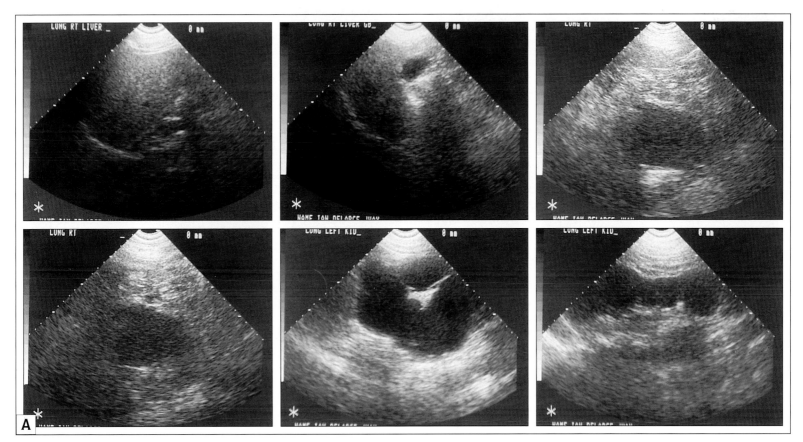

FIGURE 3-26 Polycystic kidney. Polycystic kidney disease is an autosomal dominant familial disorder leading to renal failure in adulthood. In this disorder, multiple cysts of varying size occur in the cortex and medulla, giving rise to lobulated enlargement of the kidney. Urinary tract infection frequently occurs, and when infection involves one of the cysts, it may be difficult or impossible to treat. This man aged 57 years was investigated for hypertension. Intravenous pyelogram, ultrasound, and computed tomography failed to show a right kidney. **A,** On ultrasound examination, the left kidney was large and multicystic. (*continued*)

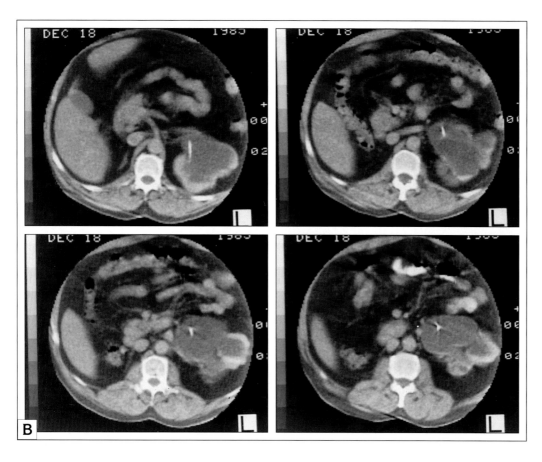

FIGURE 3-26 *(continued)* **B.** The computed tomography scan showed a large polycystic left kidney with hydronephrosis.

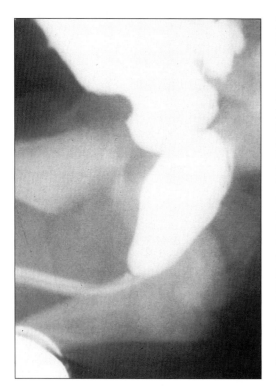

FIGURE 3-27
Posterior urethral valves. Posterior urethral valves are congenital anomalies that occur in young men, leading to obstruction and, frequently, presenting with urinary tract infection.
This voiding cysto-urethrogram from a young boy shows a posterior urethral valve with dilatation of the upper urethra and increased bladder residua. The bladder also demonstrates diverticula associated with hypertrophy and dilatation of the bladder.

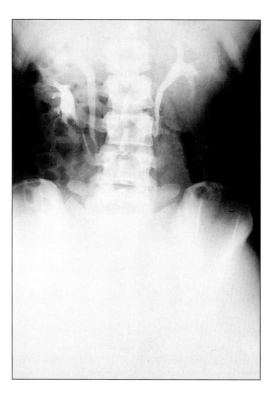

FIGURE 3-28
Duplicated collecting system. Congenital abnormalities of the genitourinary system occur frequently. One common abnormality is duplication of the collecting system. Occasionally, this may be associated with obstruction and urinary tract infection. This 17-minute intravenous pyelogram film in a woman aged 21 years who presented with pyelonephritis shows blunting and dilatation of the calyces of the upper collecting system of the duplex system on the right side.

REFLUX NEPHROPATHY

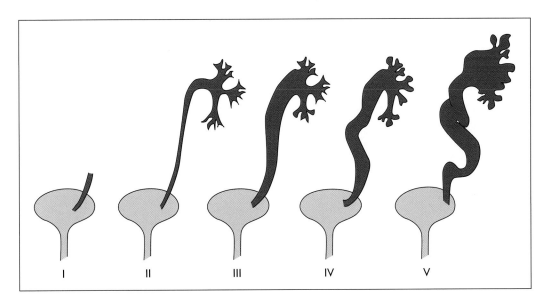

I   II   III   IV   V

FIGURE 3-29 Grades of vesicouretral reflux. Grade I reflux involves reflux of the ureter only. With grade II reflux, there is reflux of the ureter, pelvis, and calyces with no dilatation and normal calyces. In grade III, there is mild/moderate dilatation of the ureter and renal pelvis with little dilatation of the calyceal fornices. Grade IV reflux shows moderate dilatation or tortuosity of the ureter and dilatation of the pelvis and calyces, with alteration of the sharp angles of the fornices but maintenance of papillary impressions. In grade V reflux, there is gross dilatation and tortuosity of the ureter, pelvis, and calyces [9].

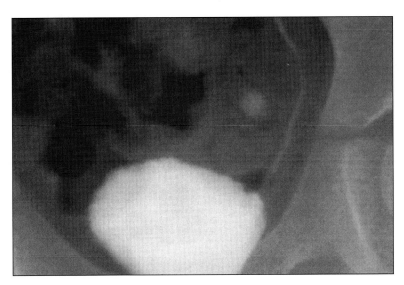

FIGURE 3-30 Grade I reflux in a voiding cystourethrogram. Some contrast is evident in the lower ureters only. Grade I reflux is common in children with urinary tract infection and generally resolves with treatment of the infection.

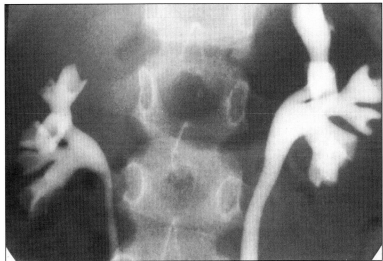

FIGURE 3-31 Grades II and III reflux in a voiding cystourethrogram from a young boy presenting with recurrent urinary tract infections. On the right side is grade II reflux, with good presentation of the calyces. Some early clubbing of the calyces and dilatation of the ureter can be seen on the left side, which is grade III reflux.

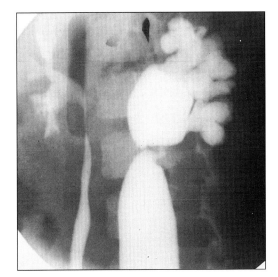

FIGURE 3-32 Grades II and IV reflux in a voiding cystourethrogram from a young boy presenting with recurrent urinary tract infections. In this case, the right side shows grade II reflux, but the left side shows grade IV reflux with massive dilatation of the upper tract and ureter.

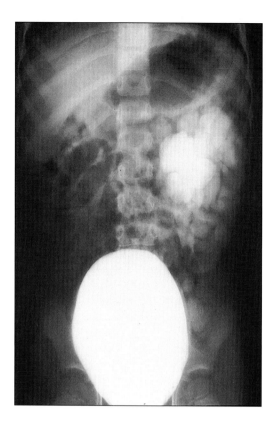

FIGURE 3-33 Voiding cystourethrogram showing grade V reflux in a boy aged 3.5 years with recurrent urinary tract infections. The voiding cystourethrogram shows a hugely dilated left renal pelvis and calyces, with destruction of the calyceal architecture. The ureter is tortuous and grossly dilated.

OTHER INFECTIONS

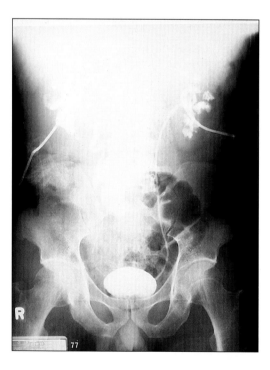

FIGURE 3-34 Renal tuberculosis. Tuberculosis of the urinary tract may lead to extensive abnormalities and destruction of renal tissue. This woman aged 33 years had a 6-month history of illness and presented with renal failure. Her urine was found to be positive for *Mycobacterium tuberculosis*. She subsequently had bilateral nephrostomy tubes and a left ureteric stent placed. This radiograph shows bilateral nephrotomograms. On the right side, there is severe clubbing of the interpolar calyces and multiple filling defects in the calyces, which are themselves irregular and inflamed. Similarly, in the left kidney, there are gross calyceal changes. The irregularity of the involved calyces is similar to papillary necrosis from other causes. There are bilateral changes in the ureters associated with tuberculosis as well, with multiple ulcerations causing a ragged, irregular appearance of the ureteral wall. With healing, there are multiple areas of ureteral strictures alternating with dilated segments to produce a beaded or corkscrew appearance.

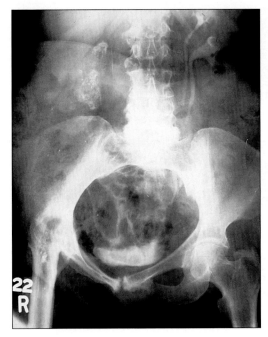

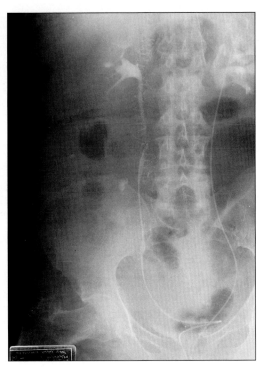

FIGURE 3-36 Renal candidiasis. Renal candidiasis results from hematogenous spread from skin or lung infection or from ascension of yeast from the bladder. This retrograde pyelogram, obtained from a diabetic woman aged 75 years with previous urinary tract infection with *Proteus mirabilis* and *Escherichia coli*, demonstrates moderate hydronephrosis on the left with abnormal upper pole calyces. Characteristically, with renal candidiasis, there are shaggy irregular filling defects in the renal pelvis due to rapidly growing hyphal masses. These masses may obstruct the collecting system and cause renal colic. Untreated, candidiasis may result in acute papillary necrosis or chronic pyelonephritis with renal failure.

FIGURE 3-35 Intravenous pyelogram showing autonephrectomy in renal tuberculosis. In advanced stages of renal tuberculosis, an autonephrectomy occurs with complete loss of function of the involved kidney. This intravenous pyelogram shows calcification of a nonfunctioning right kidney in a woman with tuberculosis. Note also the left duplex collecting system. The fused right hip also is secondary to tuberculosis.

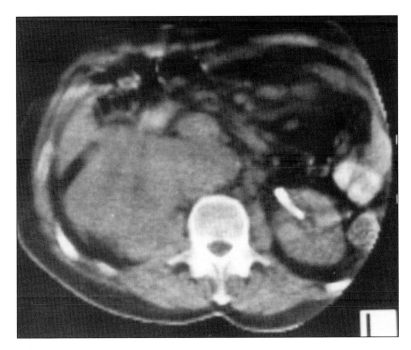

FIGURE 3-37 *Candida albicans* pyelonephritis. This computed tomography scan in a patient with candidal infection of the kidney shows that the entire right kidney has been replaced by an inflammatory renal mass, secondary to *C. albicans* infection.

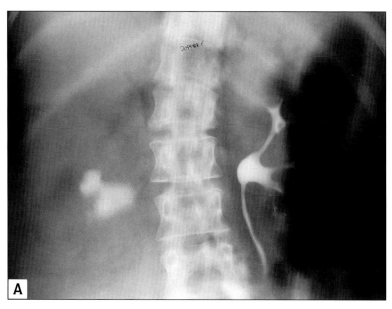

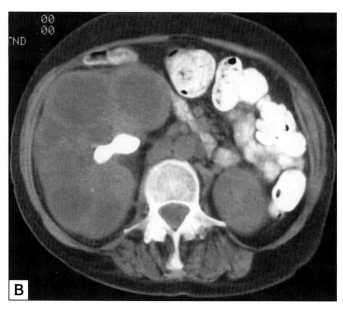

FIGURE 3-38 Xanthogranulomatous pyelonephritis. Xanthogranulomatous pyelonephritis is a rare disease associated with *Escherichia coli* or *Proteus mirabilis* infection, with replacement of the renal parenchyma by an inflammatory mass. **A,** Tomogram of a patient with right-sided xanthogranulomatous pyelonephritis. The left calyces are normal, except for minor blunting inferiorly, but the right kidney shows only a collection of contrast material where the renal pelvis should be. **B,** The computed tomography scan shows replacement of the right kidney by a huge multilobulated inflammatory mass. *P. mirabilis* was grown from the urine of this patient.

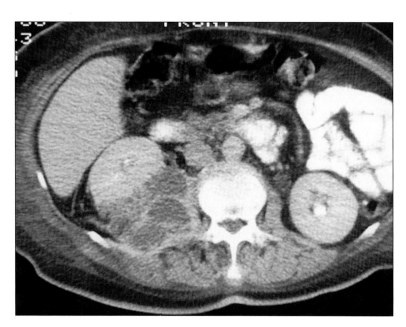

FIGURE 3-39 Abdominal computed tomography scan showing xanthogranulomatous pyelonephritis due to *Escherichia coli.* Computed tomography scan shows a large multiloculated mass in the area of the right kidney, with displacement of kidney tissue laterally and superiorly. There is a small amount of contrast material present in the remnant of the renal pelvis.

PREGNANCY

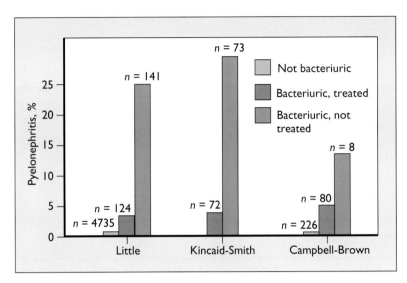

FIGURE 3-40 Pyelonephritis in pregnancy. Women with asymptomatic bacteriuria early in pregnancy have a high risk of pyelonephritis later in the pregnancy (end of the second trimester or early third trimester) if untreated. This increased occurrence of pyelonephritis is likely secondary to the physiologic hydronephrosis and obstruction associated with pregnancy. Treatment of asymptomatic bacteriuria decreases the risk of subsequent pyelonephritis tenfold. Studies reporting pyelonephritis in women identified with asymptomatic bacteriuria early in pregnancy and subsequently randomized to treatment or nontreatment are summarized in this figure. The risk of pyelonephritis is approximately 30% for women identified with asymptomatic bacteriuria in early pregnancy who are not treated [10–12].

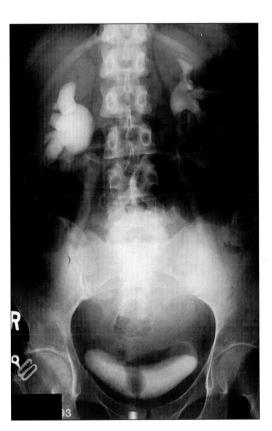

FIGURE 3-41 Intravenous pyelogram demonstrating physiologic hydronephrosis during pregnancy. Physiologic hormonal changes cause dilatation of the genitourinary system, and the enlarging uterine mass may cause extrinsic pressure on the ureter, leading to progressive dilatation of the proximal collecting system. The dilatation usually is more prominent and develops earlier on the right side. Following delivery, the urinary tract returns to normal within several weeks. This intravenous pyelogram was obtained from a P3 G3 woman aged 23 years with hematuria 2 days postpartum. No cause for the hematuria is seen in the pyelogram, but it demonstrates the moderate dilatation of both kidneys and ureters associated with pregnancy. This physiologic hydronephrosis is believed to be responsible for the increased occurrence of pyelonephritis in pregnancy in women with asymptomatic bacteriuria.

Asymptomatic bacteriuria in pregnancy: When to screen?
12–16 weeks' gestation
Use culture method
If negative, no further screening generally recommended
Consider second screening at 20–24 wks for women with history of prior recurrent urinary tract infection

FIGURE **3-42** When to screen for asymptomatic bacteriuria in pregnancy.

Risks of asymptomatic bacteriuria in pregnancy
Well-documented
Acute pyelonephritis
Probable
Low birth weight
Premature labor and delivery
Stillbirth

FIGURE **3-43** Risks of asymptomatic bacteriuria in pregnancy.

REFERENCES

1. Rubin RH, Shapiro ED, Andriole VT, *et al.*: Evaluation of new anti-infective drugs for the treatment of urinary infection. *Clin Infect Dis* 1992, 15:S216–S227.

2. Louie TJ, Nicolle L, Dubois J, *et al.*: Randomized comparison of lomefloxacin and trimethoprim-sulfamethoxazole for the treatment of complicated urinary tract infections [abstract 131]. Presented at the 30th annual meeting of the Interscience Conference on Antimicrobial Agents and Chemotherapy, 1990.

3. Cox EC: A comparison of the safety and efficacy of lomefloxacin and ciprofloxacin in the treatment of complicated or recurrent urinary tract infections. *Am J Med* 1992, 92:82S–86S.

4. Waites KB, Cannupp KC, DeVivo MJ: Epidemiology and risk factors for urinary tract infection following spinal cord injury. *Arch Phys Med Rehabil* 1993, 74:691–695.

5. Vejlsgaard R: Studies on urinary infection in diabetics: I. Bacteriuria in patients with diabetes mellitus and in control subjects. *Acta Med Scand* 1966, 179:173–182.

6. Ooi BS, Chen BTM, Yu M: Prevalence and site of bacteriuria in diabetes mellitus. *Postgrad Med J* 1974, 50:497–499.

7. Jaspan JB, Mangera C, Krut LH: Bacteriuria in black diabetics. *S Afr Med J* 1977, 51:374–376.

8. Schmitt JK, Fawcett CJ, Gullickson G: Asymptomatic bacteriuria and hemoglobin. *Diabetes Care* 1986, 9:518–520.

9. Report of the International Reflux Study Committee: Medical versus surgical treatment of primary vesicoureteral reflux. *Pediatrics* 1981, 67:392.

10. Little PJ: The incidence of urinary infection in 5,000 pregnant women. *Lancet* 1966, 2:925–928.

11. Kincaid-Smith P, Bullen M: Bacteriuria in pregnancy. *Lancet* 1965, i:395–399.

12. Campbell-Brown M, McFadyen R, Seal DJ, Stephenson ML: Is screening for bacteriuria in pregnancy worthwhile? *BMJ* 1987, 294:1579–1582.

SELECTED BIBLIOGRAPHY

Patterson TF, Andriole VT: Bacteriuria in pregnancy. *Infect Dis Clin North Am* 1987, 1:807–822.

Report of the International Reflux Study Committee: Medical versus surgical treatment of primary vesicoureteral reflux. *Pediatrics* 1981, 67:392.

Rubin RH, Shapiro ED, Andriole VT, *et al.*: Evaluation of new anti-infective drugs for the treatment of urinary infection. *Clin Infect Dis* 1992, 15:S216–S227.

Waites KB, Cannupp KC, DeVivo MJ: Epidemiology and risk factors for urinary tract infection following spinal cord injury. *Arch Phys Med Rehabil* 1993, 74:691–695.

Zhanel G, Harding GKM, Nicolle LE: Asymptomatic bacteriuria in diabetics. *Rev Infect Dis* 1991, 13:150–154.

CHAPTER 4

Infections of the Prostate

Edward D. Kim
Anthony J. Schaeffer

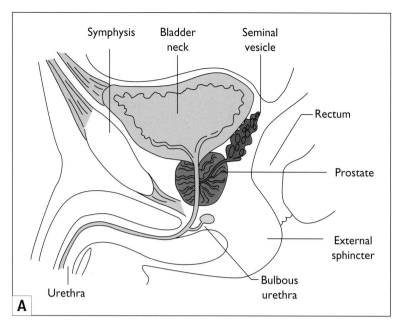

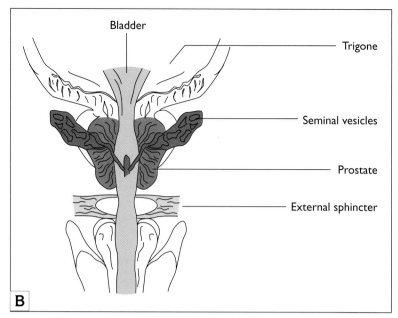

FIGURE 4-1 Anatomy of the prostate. **A,** Coronal view. **B,** Sagittal view. The prostate gland is an accessory sex gland, providing approximately 15% of the ejaculate. The base of the prostate abuts the bladder neck, whereas the apex is in continuity with the membranous urethra, resting on the urogenital diaphragm. The adult prostate weighs approximately 20 g, but may increase in size dramatically with age. The approximate dimensions are 4.4 cm transversely at the base, 3.4 cm in length, and 2.6 cm in anteroposterior diameter. Antibacterial factors, such as zinc, within the prostate help to prevent infection.

Classification of prostatitis

Acute bacterial prostatitis: Acute bacterial infection of prostate gland accompanied by systemic constitutional and local signs of infection, pyuria, and bacteriuria

Chronic bacterial prostatitis: Chronic persistent bacterial process in absence of systemic and infrequent local symptoms, usually presenting with recurrent symptomatic episodes of bacteriuria

Nonbacterial prostatitis: Inflammatory syndrome indistinguishable from chronic bacterial prostatitis that similarly presents with pyuria, but no typical uropathogens are cultured in prostatic secretions and urine

Prostatodynia: Devoid of objective manifestations of prostatic urinary tract inflammation or evidence of infection; clinically, local symptoms are common and simulate prostatic inflammation

---

FIGURE 4-2 Classification of prostatitis. Up to an estimated 50% of men will experience prostate-related voiding symptoms at some point in their lives [1]. Although the relative incidence of the various types of prostatitis have not been well characterized, in one study of 600 men at a special prostatitis clinic, most men had nonbacterial prostatitis [2]. Acute bacterial prostatitis is a very uncommon occurrence, even in comparison with chronic bacterial prostatitis.

Types of prostatitis, by EPS and culture

Classification	EPS	Culture (EPS)	Rectal examination
Acute bacterial prostatitis	↑ PMNs* (++++)	Positive—Enterobacteriaceae	Exquisitely tender
Chronic bacterial prostatitis	↑ PMNs (++)	Positive—Enterobacteriaceae	Normal
Nonbacterial prostatitis	↑ PMNs (++)	Absent bacteria (sterile)	Normal
Prostatodynia	Normal	Sterile	Variable

*EPS contraindicated in acute bacterial prostatitis; urine examination will provide diagnosis (pyuria, bacteriuria).

EPS—expressed prostatic secretions; PMNs—polymorphonuclear cells.

FIGURE 4-3 Types of prostatitis, by expressed prostatic secretions (EPS) and culture. The various prostatitis syndromes have been classified based on EPS and urine culture findings. This classification system is important for therapy, because the various categories are treated differently. The presence of ≥ 10 leukocytes per high-power field (hpf) in the EPS is considered clinically significant inflammation [3]. The procedure for obtaining the EPS is detailed in Figure 4-28. In acute bacterial prostatitis (ABP), EPS (as obtained by massage) should not be obtained for risk of precipitating bacteremia. If EPS is obtained inadvertently, sheets of leukocytes (polymorphonuclear cells) are present. Significant bacterial growth is present in the voided urine due to the presence of an accompanying cystitis. In chronic bacterial prostatitis, the EPS is usually associated with ≥ 10 leukocytes/hpf and should be obtained. Unlike patients with ABP, these patients are not acutely ill. Urine culture shows no growth unless the patient develops an acute urinary tract infection, in which case culture would demonstrate the same spectrum of organisms as in ABP. With nonbacterial prostatitis, significant inflammation is present in the prostate as characterized by ≥ 10 leukocytes/hpf. However, routine bacterial culture does not demonstrate growth of organisms. Cultures for fungi, *Chlamydia*, *Ureaplasma*, and *Mycoplasma* rarely demonstrate growth. In prostatodynia, no inflammation in the EPS or bacterial growth in culture is present. "Pelviperineal pain" is an appropriate name to describe the symptoms in this condition.

Possible routes of infection in prostatic infection

Ascending urethral infection
Reflux of infected urine into prostatic ducts
Migration of rectal bacteria via direct extension or
 lymphogenous spread
Hematogenous infection
Postinstrumentation

FIGURE 4-4 Possible routes of infection in prostatic infection. The actual routes of prostatic infection are unknown in most cases, but various etiologies may be found. Ascending urethral infection is a known route because of the frequency of previous gonococcal prostatitis in the past, as well as the finding of identical prostatic fluid and vaginal culture organisms in many studied couples [1]. Intraprostatic urinary reflux has been demonstrated in human cadavers and may play a role [4].

ACUTE BACTERIAL PROSTATITIS

A. Clinical manifestations of acute bacterial prostatitis: Symptoms

Manifestation	Frequency
Fever	+++
Pain, perineal discomfort	++
Dysuria	+++
Urinary frequency and urgency	+++
Urinary retention	+
Generalized malaise	++

B. Clinical manifestations of acute bacterial prostatitis: Signs

Manifestation	Frequency
Prostatic enlargement	++
Tenderness	+++
Induration	++
Firmness	++
Pyuria	+++

FIGURE 4-5 Clinical manifestations of acute bacterial prostatitis. **A.** Symptoms. Acute prostatitis is characterized by the sudden onset of symptoms, resulting in a very ill-appearing patient. Although dysuria, urgency, frequency, and fever are constant, varying degrees of bladder outlet obstruction and low back/perineal pain may be present. These fulminant symptoms may be preceded by vague pelvic and systemic manifestations for days to weeks.

B. Signs. Firm rectal palpation should be avoided in the patient with suspected acute prostatitis because of the possibility of systemically disseminating bacteria (bacteremia). A gentle digital rectal examination should be performed to assess for the possibility of an abscess, but a massage for expressed prostatic fluid has no place in the evaluation. Pyuria always accompanies an untreated acute bacterial prostatitis.

Clinical complications of acute bacterial prostatitis

Prostatic abscess
Urinary retention
Sepsis
Acute bacterial epididymitis
Chronic bacterial prostatitis

FIGURE 4-6 Clinical complications of acute bacterial prostatitis. With prompt recognition and treatment of the acute process, serious complications are uncommon. This fulminant process can lead to sepsis and death if it is not recognized quickly. Those men with benign prostatic hyperplasia are especially susceptible to developing urinary retention. All men must be considered at risk for developing chronic bacterial prostatitis, especially if treatment has been inadequate [5].

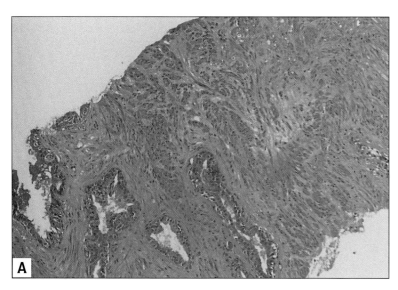

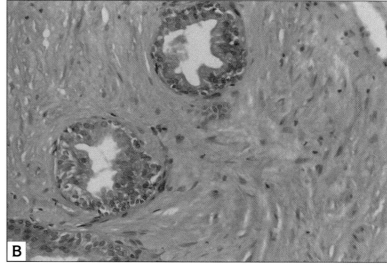

FIGURE 4-7 **A** and **B.** Histologic appearance of normal prostate tissue. Microscopic sections of normal prostate tissue, obtained by needle biopsy, show an absence of an inflammatory cell response and the preservation of stromal and ductal architecture. (Hematoxylin-eosin stain; *panel 7A,* × 40; *panel 7B,* × 100.)

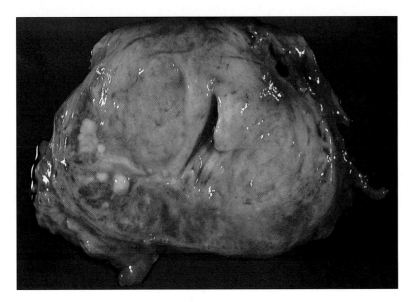

FIGURE 4-8 Gross view of acute prostatitis from an autopsy specimen. Acute prostatitis can be lethal, especially in elderly or debilitated hosts, if sepsis ensues. An enlarged, inflamed prostate with small abscesses is shown.

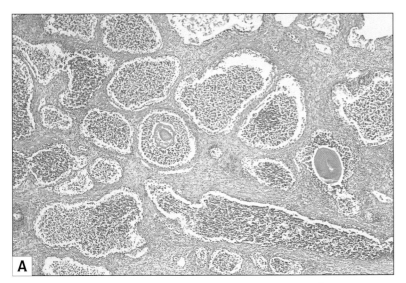

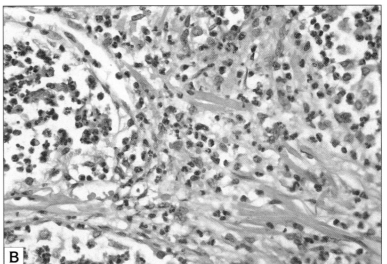

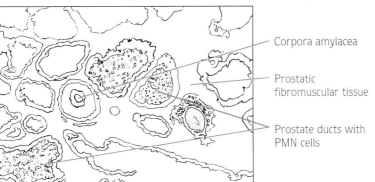

Corpora amylacea

Prostatic fibromuscular tissue

Prostate ducts with PMN cells

FIGURE 4-9 Histologic findings in acute bacterial prostatitis. **A,** Marked dilation of the prostatic ducts with polymorphonuclear (PMN) cells is seen. Incidental corpora amylacea are also present. **B,** High-power view of acute prostatitis shows marked PMN cell response in the prostatic stoma as well as in the ducts.

Diagnosis of acute bacterial prostatitis

Prompt recognition of clinical symptoms and signs
Urinalysis
Urine culture
No role for expressed prostatic secretions

FIGURE 4-10 Diagnosis of acute bacterial prostatitis. The diagnosis is based on clinical recognition of the symptoms and signs. The urine microscopic examination and urine culture are confirmatory but important components of the evaluation. The urinalysis demonstrates > 10 leukocytes per high-power field because involvement of the bladder urine is characteristic. Culture of the urine identifies the pathogenic organism and guides therapy. Because of the significant risk of bacteremia, expressed prostatic secretions should not be obtained.

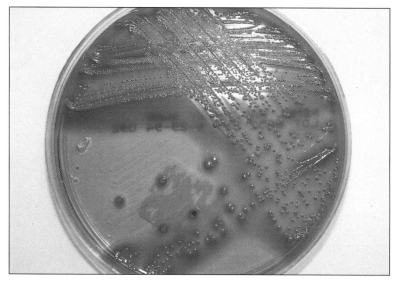

FIGURE 4-11 Urine culture in acute bacterial prostatitis showing > 10^5 colony-forming units per mL of *Escherichia coli*. *E. coli* is the most common pathogen grown in culture in acute and chronic prostatitis. *Klebsiella* and *Proteus* species are also commonly found. The clinical presentation of acute prostatitis is dramatic, often with fevers, perineal and back pain, and voiding difficulties.

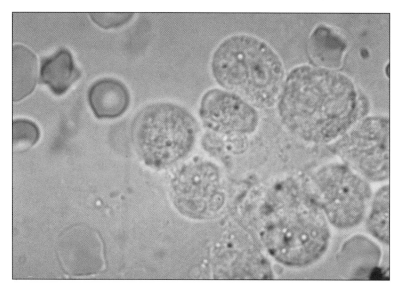

FIGURE 4-12 Pyuria in acute bacterial prostatitis. Pyuria is the presence of leukocytes in the voided urine. This inflammatory response is caused by the concurrent cystitis present in acute bacterial prostatitis. Pyuria, which is always present in untreated acute bacterial prostatitis, is not specific for this condition. The urinalysis typically demonstrates numerous leukocytes per high-power field.

Bacteriology of acute bacterial prostatitis

Escherichia coli	80%
Klebsiella spp	
Enterobacter spp	
Proteus spp	20%
Enterococcus spp	
Pseudomonas aeruginosa	
Other	

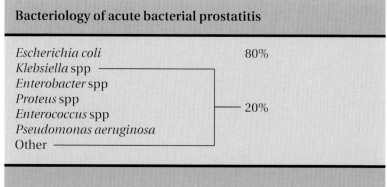

FIGURE 4-13 Bacteriology of acute bacterial prostatitis. Although most acute bacterial prostatitis is caused by *Escherichia coli*, other gram-negative enteric organisms are common causes [6]. Most investigators believe that staphylococcal and streptococcal species are uncommon causes of acute prostatitis, and instead, these organisms likely represent commensal urethral flora [1,7]. *Neisseria gonorrhoeae* was a common cause in the preantibiotic era but is rare now.

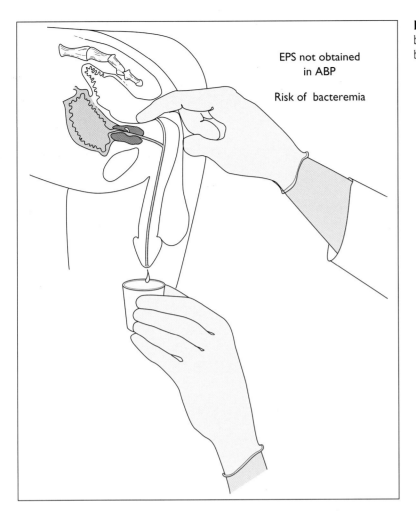

FIGURE 4-14 No expressed prostatic secretions (EPS) in acute bacterial prostatitis (ABP). Because of the significant risk of bacteremia, EPS should not be obtained in patients with ABP.

EPS not obtained in ABP

Risk of bacteremia

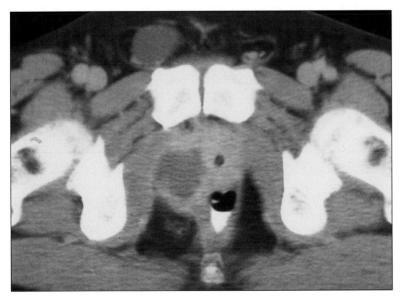

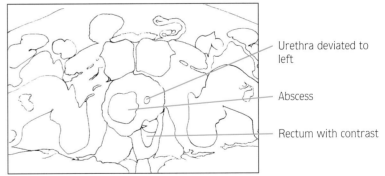

Urethra deviated to left

Abscess

Rectum with contrast

FIGURE 4-15 Computed tomography scan demonstrating a prostatic abscess. Patients with diabetes, indwelling urinary catheters, immunocompromised status, and urinary tract instrumentation and who are on maintenance hemodialysis are espe-cially prone to the development of prostatic abscess. Clinical symptoms include acute urinary retention, fever, dysuria, urinary frequency, and perineal pain. *Escherichia coli* is the predominant organism identified.

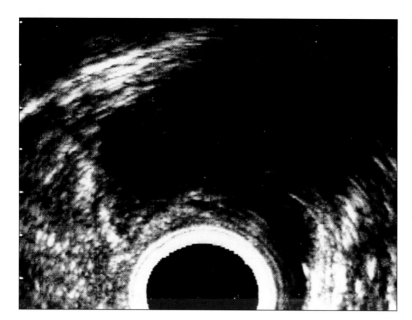

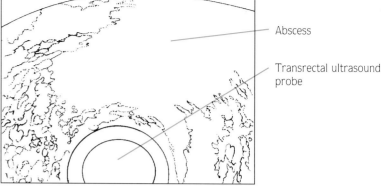

FIGURE 4-16 Transrectal ultrasound demonstrating a prostatic abscess (transverse section). Computed tomography scan and transrectal ultrasound are helpful in assessing the extent and making the diagnosis of prostatic abscess. The clinical signs of prostate tenderness and fluctuation may be present in only 35% and 16% of patients, respectively.

Principles of treatment of acute bacterial prostatitis

Pretreatment urine culture
Blood cultures
Hospitalization (most patients)
Parenteral antimicrobial therapy (recommended)
Follow-up quantitative urine cultures

FIGURE 4-17 Principles of treatment of acute bacterial prostatitis. Most patients with acute bacterial prostatitis should be hospitalized, given the potential severity of the disease process. Parenteral antimicrobial agents or oral fluoroquinolones should be started immediately, but only after a voided urine culture is obtained. Because of the febrile response in patients and the risk for bacteremia and sepsis, blood cultures are highly recommended. If the patient is hospitalized, intravenous hydration should be given. Upper and lower tract imaging studies, such as an intravenous pyelogram, ultrasound, or computed tomography scan, should be considered if the patient fails to improve. Follow-up cultures are important to ensure response to antimicrobial therapy.

Principles of antimicrobial selection in acute bacterial prostatitis

Initial therapy is empiric, directed at gram-negative
  uropathogens
Selection facilitated by urine Gram stain
Subsequent therapy based on urine culture
Acutely inflamed prostate allows good penetration of most
  antimicrobials

FIGURE 4-18 Principles of antimicrobial selection in acute bacterial prostatitis. Initial empiric therapy with an aminoglycoside and ampicillin usually results in defervescence and improvement within 48 hours. The aminoglycoside treats the enteric gram-negative organisms, whereas ampicillin treats enterococci. If the patient remains ill, a computed tomography scan of the abdomen and pelvis will evaluate for upper tract obstruction or a prostatic abscess. When the patient improves, oral antimicrobial therapy may be instituted based on susceptibility testing. Unlike the case with chronic bacterial prostatitis, most antimicrobial agents can penetrate into the prostatic tissue in the acutely inflamed state.

Empiric antimicrobial regimens for acute bacterial prostatitis

Ampicillin IV (1–2 g every 6 hrs) + gentamicin IV (1.7 mg/kg every 8 hrs)
  or
Fluoroquinolones (*eg*, ciprofloxacin 400 mg IV every 12 hrs,
  ofloxacin 200 mg IV every 12 hrs)
  or
Trimethoprim-sulfamethoxasole (IV 160/800 mg twice daily)

IV—intravenously.

FIGURE 4-19 Empiric antimicrobial regimens for acute bacterial prostatitis. Those patients appearing significantly ill, or with evidence of bacteremia or significant voiding problems, should be hospitalized and started on an aminoglycoside-penicillin derivate immediately. Usually, ampicillin and gentamicin are given, but vancomycin may be substituted for the penicillin-allergic patient. The gentamicin dosage should be adjusted according to creatinine clearance. As a second choice, a fluoroquinolone or trimethoprim-sulfamethoxasole regimen may be started until urine culture results become available. These two classes of agents are lipid-soluble and able to achieve significant concentrations within the prostate.

Duration of treatment in acute bacterial prostatitis

Minimum 4 wks recommended
Total duration controversial
After clinical improvement on parenteral therapy, switch to oral
Bacterial localization cultures recommended for recurrent or
  persistent bacteruria after therapy

FIGURE 4-20 Duration of treatment in acute bacterial prostatitis. Although the optimal duration of antimicrobial therapy is not known, a minimum 4-week regimen is recommended. Because all patients should be considered at risk for the development of chronic bacterial prostatitis, and because the diffusion of antimicrobial agents may be optimal during the period of resolution, full-dose therapy is advised. Complete bacterial localization studies at 1, 4, and 12 weeks after completion of therapy are recommended because prolonged antimicrobial treatment is required if persistence of prostatic bacteria is documented in patients with recurrent or chronic bacteruria.

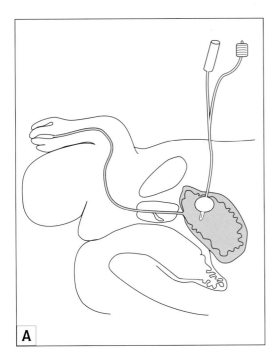 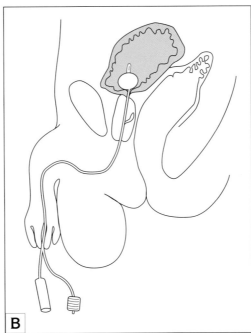

A   B

FIGURE 4-21 Principle of management of urinary obstruction. Urinary retention is not uncommon in men with concomitant benign prostatic hypertrophy. **A**, Treatment with suprapubic catheterization with a percutaneous cystostomy is recommended to avoid further trauma to the prostate. **B**, A urethral catheter may cause bacteremia from the trauma of insertion through the prostate and may impair the egress of prostatic secretions, thereby exacerbating the prostatic inflammation.

Management of prostatic abscess

Presence suspected by:
  Fluctuance on rectal examination
  Poor response to antimicrobial agents
Presence confirmed by computed tomography or ultrasound
Drainage is essential:
  Transperineal, ultrasound-guided
  Transurethral

FIGURE 4-22 Management of prostatic abscess. Although prostate abscesses are uncommon, the presence of fluctuance on the rectal examination or a poor response to antimicrobial agents should prompt further investigation. The computed tomography scan is an excellent imaging modality for diagnosis. Prompt drainage as well as parenteral antimicrobial agents are the mainstays of therapy. Drainage may be performed transperineally using transrectal ultrasound guidance or transurethrally, especially if the abscess is located centrally.

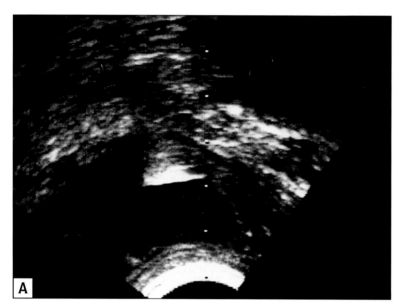

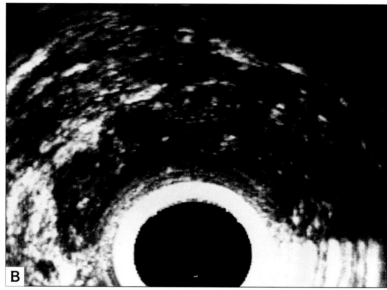

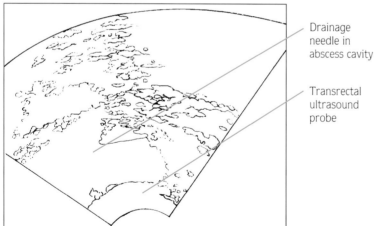

Drainage needle in abscess cavity

Transrectal ultrasound probe

FIGURE 4-23 Technique of transrectal ultrasound (TRUS)-guided drainage. The transrectal ultrasound probe is inserted gently into the rectum. Both transverse and sagittal images can define the abscess. The perineum is sterilely prepped, and a needle introduced into the prostate. The needle is inserted into the abscess under direct visual control.

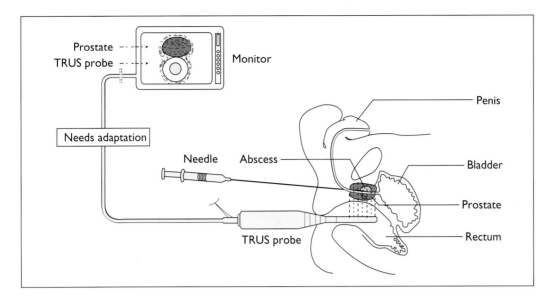

FIGURE 4-24 Technique of transrectal ultrasound (TRUS)-guided drainage. The transrectal ultrasound probe is inserted gently into the rectum. Both transverse and sagittal images can define the abscess. The perineum is sterilely prepped, and a needle introduced into the prostate. The needle is inserted into the abscess under direct visual control.

CHRONIC BACTERIAL PROSTATITIS

Chronic bacterial prostatitis: Definition

Characterized by relapsing urinary tract infections
Symptoms occasionally consist of irritative voiding symptoms and discomfort
EPS usually contains ≥ 10 leukocytes per high-power field
Urine and EPS cultures yield bacterial growth

EPS—expressed prostatic secretion.

FIGURE 4-25 Definition of chronic bacterial prostatitis. Chronic bacterial prostatitis must be demonstrated by bacterial growth in culture of prostatic fluid or postmassage urine specimen. The expressed prostatic secretions usually show ≥ 10 leukocytes per high-power field and macrophages. The hallmark finding is the occurrence of relapsing urinary tract infections, most often by the same pathogen.

Cardinal clinical manifestations of chronic bacterial prostatitis

Most common cause of relapsing urinary tract infection in men
Asymptomatic periods between episodes of recurrent bacteriuria
Obstruction or irritative voiding symptoms (occasional)
Vague discomfort in pelvis and perineum (infrequent)
Physical findings on palpation normal
Expressed prostatic secretions or postmassage urine culture needed for precise diagnosis

FIGURE 4-26 Cardinal clinical manifestations of chronic bacterial prostatitis. Relapsing urinary tract infections, with asymptomatic periods between, are common in chronic bacterial prostatitis. Although some men are diagnosed because of asymptomatic bacteriuria, most have varying degrees of irritative voiding symptoms, such as dysuria, frequency, and urgency. In addition, feelings of vague discomfort in the pelvis and perineum may be present. Fevers and chills are uncommon. Rectal palpation of the prostate is not painful and has no specific findings. Prostatic fluid and postmassage urine cultures, which should be obtained for precise diagnosis, demonstrate bacterial growth.

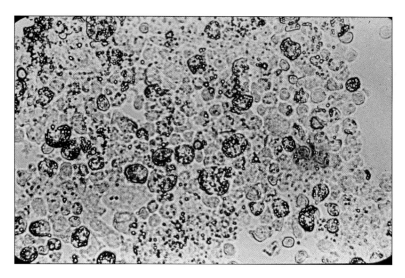

FIGURE 4-27 Use of expressed prostatic secretions in the diagnosis of chronic bacterial prostatitis. Clinically significant inflammation is considered to be present when the expressed prostatic secretions contain > 10 leukocytes per high-power field. Only 5% to 10% of men without clinical symptoms or other signs of prostatic inflammation will have such leukocyte counts.

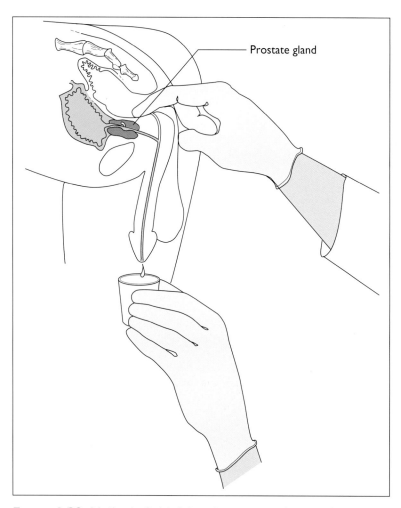

Prostate gland

FIGURE 4-28 Method of obtaining the expressed prostatic secretions (EPS). Careful technique is essential to avoid contamination in obtaining the EPS. The foreskin is retracted and the glans cleaned with tapwater prior to collection of the EPS in a sterile container. The prostate is digitally massaged from lateral to medial and then from base (superior) to apex (inferior).

Prostatic specimens: Ejaculate vs expressed prostatic secretions

Expressed prostatic secretions
Ejaculate may represent:
    Testicular colonization
    Epididymal colonization
    Seminal vesicular colonization
Ejaculate not specific for prostate

FIGURE 4-29 Use of expressed prostatic specimens versus ejaculate as prostatic specimens. Ejaculate is not as specific as the expressed prostatic secretions, because the former also contains contributions from the seminal vesicles, testes, and epididymides.

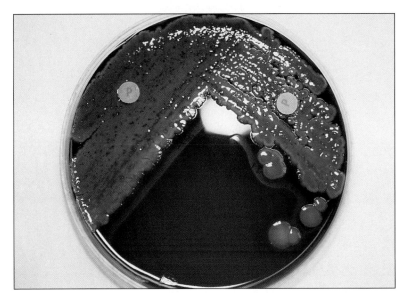

FIGURE 4-30 Urine culture with $> 10^5$ colony-forming units per mL of *Pseudomonas aeruginosa* in chronic bacterial prostatitis. Chronic bacterial prostatitis is the most common cause of relapsing urinary tract infections in men. Bacterial pathogens are essentially the same as those seen in acute prostatitis. *Pseudomonas* species and *Enterococcus* are less common than the Enterobacteriaceae. The clinical presentation is characterized by asymptomatic periods between episodes of recurrent bacteriuria. Obstructive or irritative voiding symptoms and often a vague discomfort in the pelvis and perineum are characteristic findings.

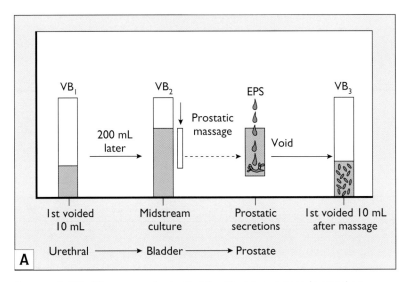

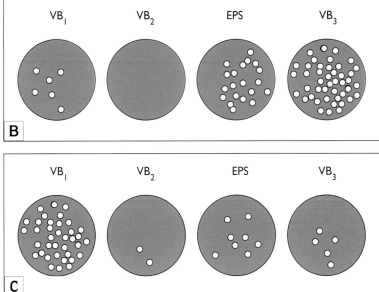

FIGURE 4-31 Three-cup test. **A**, The three-cup test is used to localize pathogenic bacteria to the prostate. The patient is instructed to void the first 10 mL of urine (VB_1), representing a urethral specimen, into a collection cup. A midstream urine specimen (VB_2), representing bladder urine, is then collected after the patient voids approximately 200 mL. After the patient empties his bladder, expressed prostatic secretions (EPS) are obtained after prostate massage. The first 10 mL of urine to be voided after prostate massage is designated VB_3 and represents prostatic washout. **B**, The VB_1, VB_2, EPS, and VB_3 are cultured. The presence of bacteria in the EPS or VB_3 culture when the VB_1 and VB_2 show no growth is highly diagnostic for bacterial prostatitis. Also, a tenfold higher number of colony-forming units per mL from the EPS and VB_3 when compared with the VB_1 and VB_2 are indicative of bacterial prostatitis. **C**, Growth of gram-negative bacilli from VB_1 without significant growth in the remainder of the differential cultures is diagnostic of urethral colonization. Gram-positive staphylococcal and streptococcal species frequently colonize the distal urethra and do not cause bacterial prostatitis [8].

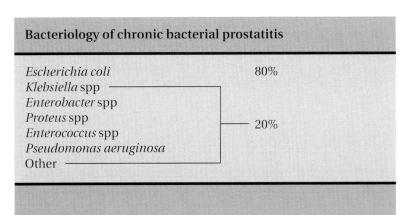

Bacteriology of chronic bacterial prostatitis	
Escherichia coli	80%
Klebsiella spp	
Enterobacter spp	
Proteus spp	20%
Enterococcus spp	
Pseudomonas aeruginosa	
Other	

FIGURE 4-32 Bacteriology of chronic bacterial prostatitis. The spectrum of organisms grown in culture in chronic bacterial prostatitis is essentially the same as that in acute bacterial prostatitis. Most infections are caused by a single pathogen, but a polymicrobial infection is not unusual. Obligate anaerobic bacteria rarely cause prostatic infection. Localization cultures need not demonstrate $> 100,000$ colony-forming units per mL for the diagnosis, but rather the presence of a $>$ tenfold bacterial growth in the expressed prostatic secretions or VB_3 specimen is important [9].

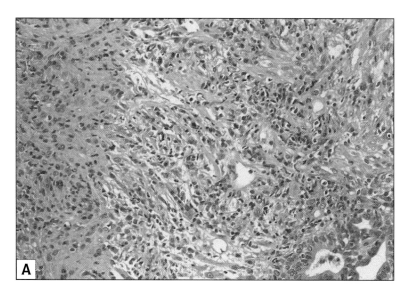
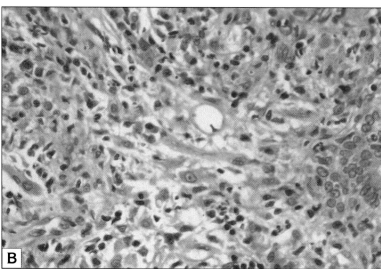

FIGURE 4-33 Histologic findings in chronic bacterial prostatitis. **A**, Microscopic section of chronic prostatitis shows a nonspecific mixed inflammatory infiltrate consisting of lymphocytes, plasma cells, and histiocytes. **B**, High-power view of chronic prostatitis. (Hematoxylin-eosin stain; *panel 33A*, × 40; *panel 33B*, × 200.)

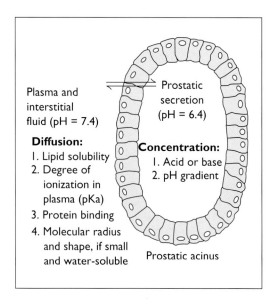

FIGURE 4-34 Factors determining diffusion and concentration of antimicrobial agents in the prostate. The reasons for relapsing urinary tract infections include the poor penetration of most antimicrobial agents into the prostatic fluid and/or bacterial sequestration, which protects them from antimicrobial exposure. Only small molecular size, un-ionized, lipid-soluble drugs not firmly bound to plasma proteins are able to diffuse across the epithelial membrane. (*Adapted from* Stamey *et al.* [10].)

Penetration of antimicrobials in chronic bacterial prostatitis

Good	Poor
Macrolides	Aminoglycosides
Trimethoprim-sulfamethoxazole	β-Lactams
Rifampin	
Fluoroquinolones	

FIGURE 4-35 Penetration of antimicrobials in chronic bacterial prostatitis. Those antimicrobial agents, such as fluoroquinolones and trimethoprim-sulfamethoxazole, which most effectively penetrate into the prostatic fluid, are good treatment choices for chronic bacterial prostatitis. Highly bactericidal activity has been demonstrated against the Enterobacteriaceae group and *Pseudomonas aeruginosa* using fluoroquinolones, a class of antimicrobial agents that inhibits bacterial DNA replication and protein synthesis. Fluoroquinolones are generally ineffective against the streptococci, including enterococci, and anaerobes. Penicillin derivates are generally ineffective in treating this condition. The treatment of chronic bacterial prostatitis is based on urine and expressed prostatic secretion culture results.

Recommended antimicrobial regimens for chronic bacterial prostatitis	
Agent	**Dosage regimen**
Trimethoprim-sulfamethoxazole	160 mg/800 mg po bid × 12 wks
Fluoroquinolone	
Ciprofloxacin	500 mg po bid × 12 wks
Ofloxacin	400 mg po bid × 12 wks

bid—twice daily; po—orally.

FIGURE 4-36 Recommended antimicrobial regimens for chronic bacterial prostatitis. Trimethoprim-sulfamethoxazole has been the single drug studied most extensively in this condition. Meares' studies have demonstrated a 15% cure rate with 2 weeks of full-dose oral therapy [11], whereas cure rates of 40% have been achieved with a 12-week course of therapy. The standard oral dosage is one double-strength tablet (160 mg trimethoprim/800 mg sulfamethoxazole) twice daily. More recent studies using fluoroquinolones have demonstrated bacteriologic cure rates of 54% to 92% [12]. For this reason, we initially prescribe a fluoroquinolone such as noroxin (400 mg twice daily), ciprofloxacin (500 mg twice daily), ofloxacin (200–300 mg twice daily), or enoxacin (200 mg twice daily). Treatment should be continued for a minimum of 6 weeks and for up to 12 weeks if well tolerated.

Treatment of recurrent bacterial prostatitis

Suppressive chronic therapy may be required
Indicated after failed full-dose, long-term treatment (12 wks)
Regimens:
  Trimethoprim-sulfamethoxazole, 80 mg/400 mg once daily
  Nitrofurantoin, 100 mg once daily

FIGURE 4-37 Treatment of recurrent bacterial prostatitis. Suppressive antimicrobial therapy may be used to manage those patients not cured with full-dose treatment. The agent used should be selected on the basis of the susceptibility of the pathogen known to persist in the prostate. One single-strength tablet daily of trimethoprim-sulfamethoxazole or 100 mg of nitrofurantoin once or twice daily have each been used as continuous, low-dose therapy. Fluoroquinolones, minocycline, and doxycycline may also be used. Recurrence is often inevitable after cessation of even prolonged suppressive therapy.

Role of prostatectomy in chronic bacterial prostatitis

Rarely indicated
"Radical" transurethral prostatectomy suggested
Possibly more effective in men with prostatic calculi

FIGURE 4-38 Role of prostatectomy in chronic bacterial prostatitis. The "radical" transurethral prostatectomy has been suggested as a surgical treatment for resection of all infected prostatic tissue. Because most of the inflammation is located in the peripheral zone of the gland, an extensive resection of the gland is required to remove all infected and potentially infected tissue down to the level of the true prostatic capsule. Only one series of 10 patients, most having prostatic calculi, has been reported, but all men were considered cured [13]. This procedure is indicated, although only rarely, for those men failing 1 year of medical pharmacotherapy with well-documented bacterial infections.

NONBACTERIAL PROSTATITIS

Nonbacterial prostatitis: Definition

Also called abacterial prostatitis or prostatosis
Most common prostatitis syndrome
EPS contains ≥ 10 leukocytes per high-power field
Urine and EPS culture show no growth

EPS—expressed prostatic secretion.

FIGURE 4-39 Definition of nonbacterial prostatitis. Nonbacterial prostatitis is the most common form of the prostatitis syndromes and is approximately eight times more common than bacterial prostatitis. This condition is characterized by negative bacterial cultures in the presence of ≥ 10 leukocytes per high-power field in the expressed prostatic secretions.

Clinical presentation of nonbacterial prostatitis

Irritative or obstructive voiding symptoms
May be subclinical or asymptomatic
Pain localized to pelvis, perineum, or low back
No urinary tract infections

FIGURE 4-40 Clinical presentation of nonbacterial prostatitis. The presentation of nonbacterial prostatitis is clinically similar to that of chronic bacterial prostatitis, with the exception of having no growth in the urine culture. Irritative or obstructive voiding symptoms are common, but the patient may also be asymptomatic and is detected on routine urinalysis with sterile pyuria. Pain or discomfort in the pelvis, perineum, scrotum, or low back are also seen.

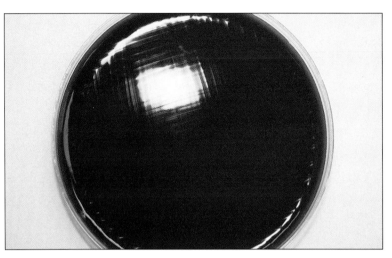

FIGURE 4-41 Blood agar culture plate with no growth in nonbacterial prostatitis. Routine urine cultures show no growth in nonbacterial prostatitis. The symptom complex and expressed prostatic secretion findings may be identical to those of chronic prostatitis, but the patient does not have a history of culture-documented urinary tract infections. The role of *Chlamydia trachomatis* and *Ureaplasma urealyticum* is equivocal.

Microbiology of nonbacterial prostatitis

Routine cultures show no growth
Specialized culture may grow
  Chlamydia or *Ureaplasma*
  Candida spp
  Blastomycoses dermatitidis
  Cryptococcus neoformans
  Histoplasma capsulatum
  Coccidioidomyces immitis
  Mycobacterium tuberculosis
  Parasites (*eg, Trichomonas vaginalis*)

FIGURE 4-42 Microbiology of nonbacterial prostatitis. The vast majority of evaluations of nonbacterial prostatitis demonstrate no growth of any organism. Prostatitis caused by *Chlamydia* and *Ureaplasma* is controversial, and these agents probably play an insignificant role in the etiology of nonbacterial cases. Prostatic involvement from the other organisms has been noted as rare case reports in the literature [14].

Chlamydia and nonbacterial prostatitis

Role is controversial
Difficulty distinguishing between urethral colonization and
  prostatic infection
Role of *Ureaplasma urealyticum* also unclear

FIGURE 4-43 *Chlamydia* and nonbacterial prostatitis. The role of *Chlamydia trachomatis* and *Ureaplasma urealyticum* is controversial in nonbacterial prostatitis. One study found that 39 of 70 men (56%) with chronic prostatitis had growth of *C. trachomatis* in the early-morning voided specimen, prostatic fluid, or seminal fluid culture, but 17% of the control population also had growth [15]. Other studies have failed to identify this organism from the prostatic fluid or to detect significant prostatic fluid antibody titers against *Chlamydia* in men with nonbacterial prostatitis [16,17]. Growth of these organisms in culture may represent urethral colonization, rather than actual prostatic infection [18,19].

Diagnosis of nonbacterial prostatitis

No documented urinary tract infections despite repeated
  cultures
Expressed prostatic secretions contain ≥ 10 leukocytes per high-
  power field
Prostate biopsy for other reasons: special stains may demonstrate rare fungal infection

FIGURE 4-44 Diagnosis of nonbacterial prostatitis. Nonbacterial prostatitis is defined as the presence of prostatic inflammation as detected on examination of the expressed prostatic secretions in the absence of positive urine cultures. A rare fungal prostatitis may be detected if a prostate biopsy is obtained for other reasons, such as an elevated serum prostate specific antigen level or abnormal digital rectal examination. A fungal culture of the expressed prostatic secretions and tissue then would be required. Routine prostate biopsy in the evaluation of nonbacterial prostatitis is not recommended.

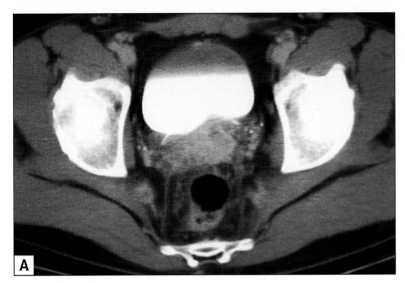

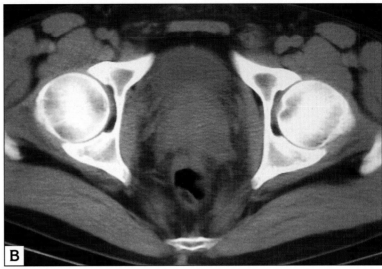

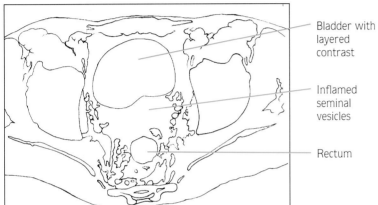

Bladder with layered contrast

Inflamed seminal vesicles

Rectum

FIGURE 4-45 Computed tomography (CT) scans in prostatic blastomycosis. **A,** CT scan of the pelvis at the level of the seminal vesicles in a patient with blastomycosis of the prostate shows prominent inflammation of the seminal vesicles. Although organisms are infrequently identified in chronic nonbacterial prostatitis, fungal infections should be considered. This patient had multiple negative bacterial cultures of the expressed prostatic secretions and urine. Persistent positive expressed prostatic secretion microscopic examinations and symptoms as well as hemospermia eventually prompted fungal cultures. **B,** CT scan of the pelvis at the level of the prostate. An enlarged prostate gland and periprostatic inflammatory changes are present.

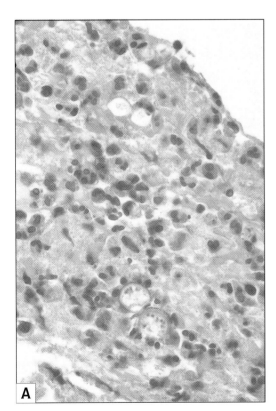

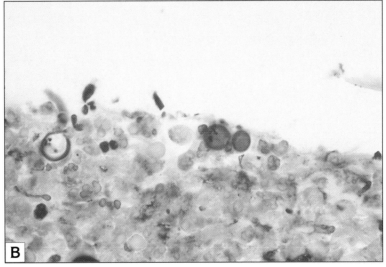

FIGURE 4-46 Histologic findings in prostatic blastomycosis. **A,** A prostate biopsy section, stained with hematoxylin-eosin, demonstrates numerous polymorphonuclear cells and several broad-based yeast buds with the characteristic doubly refractile cell wall. **B,** Gomori methenamine silver stain highlights the yeast buds. (*Courtesy of* G. Hessel, MD.)

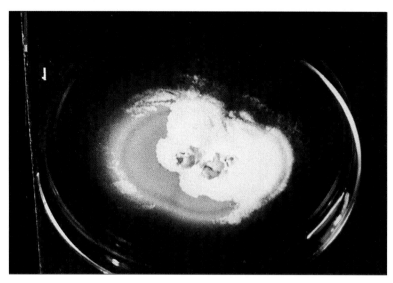

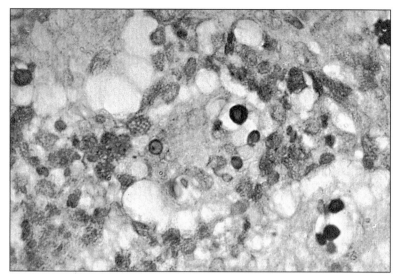

FIGURE 4-47 Fungal culture of expressed prostatic secretion fluid in prostatic blastomycosis. Blastomycosis is acquired by the inhalation of the conidia of *Blastomyces dermatitidis*. This dimorphic fungus occurs in the mycelial phase (*right*) at ambient temperatures and in the yeast phase (*left*) in the infected host or at 37° C. (*Courtesy of* G. Hessel, MD.)

FIGURE 4-48 Histologic section in cryptococcal prostatitis. Cryptococcal prostatitis is another example of a granulomatous prostatitis that is caused by *Cryptococcus neoformans*. Most cases reported have been found on postmortem examination; however, occasionally patients with AIDS are diagnosed clinically [20,21]. Genitourinary involvement with *Cryptococcus* is a manifestation of systemic disease and thus should be treated with systemic antifungal therapy. Survival in untreated patients has been poor. This section of prostate, obtained by transurethral resection, shows scattered encapsulated cryptococci in an area with multiple histiocytes. (Alcian green–periodic acid–Schiff stain.) (*From* Brock and Grieco [20]; with permission.)

Clinical presentation of granulomatous prostatitis

Specific granulomatous prostatitis
  Often present with manifestations of systemic disease
  Obstructive and irritative voiding symptom common
Nonspecific granulomatous prostatitis
  Noneosinophilic
    Acute signs and symptoms of bladder outlet obstruction
    Enlarged, firm prostate suggestive of carcinoma
  Eosinophilic
    Patients severely ill with high fevers
    Urinary retention common

FIGURE 4-49 Clinical presentation of granulomatous prostatitis. Granulomatous prostatitis may result from specific causes, such as mycotic, parasitic, or tuberculous etiologies. Patients often present with signs of disseminated disease but also may be minimally symptomatic. The nonspecific granulomatous prostatitis conditions are not commonly seen in practice but may mimic prostatic carcinoma or even acute prostatitis. The noneosinophilic type may represent a tissue response to extravasated prostatic fluid [22]. Urine cultures are sterile but occasionally may grow coliforms. The eosinophilic variety may be associated with a fibrinoid necrosis and generalized vasculitis. Also known as allergic granuloma of the prostate, complete urinary retention often develops because of the significant enlargement of the prostate.

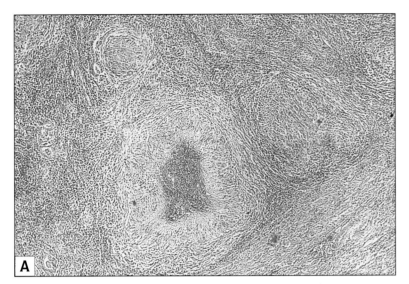

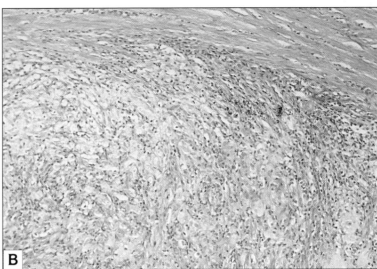

FIGURE 4-50 Histopathologic findings in granulomatous prostatitis. This condition is characterized by nodular inflammatory infiltrates composed of histiocytes, lymphocytes, and variable numbers of giant cells. Possible causes include tuberculosis, previous surgical resection, resolving acute bacterial prostatitis, and leakage of prostatic secretions into the stroma. An eosinophilic variant is also recognized. **A**, Low-power view. **B**, High-power view.

Management of fungal prostatitis
Evaluate for disseminated disease
Assess immunologic status
Antifungal therapy based on fungus isolated from expressed prostatic secretions, tissue, or urine culture
Systemic antifungal (*eg*, intravenous amphotericin B, itraconazole, or fluconazole)

FIGURE 4-51 Management of fungal prostatitis. Because of the association of fungal prostatitis with disseminated fungemia and immunocompromised states, such as AIDS or chronic steroid usage, these conditions must be evaluated carefully. Long-term treatment with systemic antifungal agents is required, following the procurement of expressed prostatic secretions, tissue, or urine fungal culture and susceptibilities. Although systemic amphotericin B has been the mainstay of therapy in the past, azole therapy with itraconazole or fluconazole is now recommended.

Management of nonfungal, nonbacterial prostatitis
Specific, reliable treatments are unavailable
Chronic antimicrobial therapy not appropriate
Doxycycline may be effective if *Chlamydia trachomatis* or *Ureaplasma urealyticum* present
Hot sitz baths, prostate massage, nonsteroidal anti-inflammatory drugs, diazepam, or anticholinergics may help relieve symptoms

FIGURE 4-52 Management of nonfungal, nonbacterial prostatitis. Because the etiology of this condition is unknown, treatment is empiric and often unrewarding. The only role for antimicrobial agents is if *Ureaplasma urealyticum* or *Chlamydia trachomatis* is suspected. Regimens include doxycycline (100 mg orally twice daily), minocycline (100 mg orally twice daily), erythromycin (500 mg four times daily × 14 days), or azolides (azithromycin, clarithromycin). Prostatic massage may be effective in men with "congested" prostates from infrequent sexual activity.

PROSTATODYNIA

Prostatodynia: Definition
Also known as pelviperineal pain
Expressed prostatic secretions are normal
Urine culture shows no growth
Functional disorder suspected from neuromuscular dysfunction of bladder outlet and prostatic urethra

FIGURE 4-53 Definition of prostatodynia. The typical patient with prostatodynia is young to middle-aged with variable signs and symptoms of abnormal urinary flow, irritative voiding dysfunction, and perineal/lower back pain. Despite symptoms that are similar to the other prostatitis syndromes, these men have normal expressed prostatic secretions and no bacterial growth in culture. Urodynamic studies have demonstrated spasm and narrowing of the urethra at the bladder neck and just proximal to the external urethral sphincter in these men, with resultant incomplete funneling. Thus, a functional disorder is suspected.

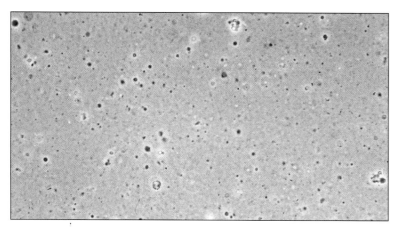

FIGURE 4-54 Expressed prostatic secretions in prostatadynia. The expressed prostatic secretions in prostatodynia, also known as pelviperineal pain, is consistently normal. Normal secretory granules of the prostate are present.

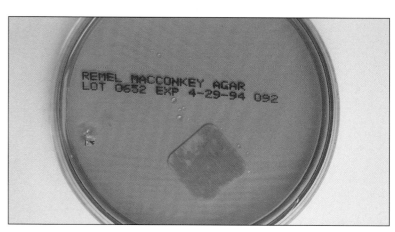

FIGURE 4-55 Urine culture in prostatodynia. Urine culture shows no growth. The typical patient is young to middle-aged with symptoms similar to those found in nonbacterial prostatitis. Stress and neuromuscular dysfunction of the bladder outlet and prostatic urethra are suspected as causative.

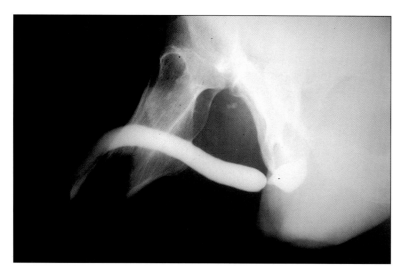

FIGURE 4-56 Retrograde urethrogram demonstrating a tight bulbous urethral stricture in a patient with prostatodynia. Anatomic causes for lower urinary tract voiding symptoms must also be suspected. This patient's stricture in the bulbar urethra was causing obstructive and irritative voiding symptoms with negative expressed prostatic secretions and urine culture.

Evaluation of the patient with prostatodynia

Expressed prostatic secretions and urine culture
Diligent history for emotional or psychosocial stresses
Consider videourodynamic studies

FIGURE 4-57 Evaluation of the patient with prostatodynia. The expressed prostatic secretions and urine cultures are essential steps to classify the patient with this disorder. A careful history should be performed for evaluating potential stressors, because many clinicians believe that psychologic factors play a primary role. Because the symptoms are probably the result of nonrelaxation and spasm of the internal urinary sphincter and pelvic floor striated muscles, videourodynamic studies may document the presence and location of the problem [23]. The physician must also be aware that conditions such as benign prostatic hypertrophy, interstitial cystitis, and carcinoma-in-situ of the bladder may present with similar complaints.

Management of prostatodynia

Selective α_1-blockers
  Prazosin
  Terazosin
Diazepam
Hot sitz baths

FIGURE 4-58 Management of prostatodynia. Treatment with the selective α_1-blockers has been effective because this class of medications serves to relax the smooth muscles of the bladder neck and prostate, which are rich in α-adrenergic receptors. Diazepam, often in combination with an α_1-blocker, is helpful in men with tension myalgia of the pelvic floor. Hot sitz baths may be used liberally. Those patients with significant emotional problems or psychosocial stressors may benefit from a psychologic or psychiatric evaluation.

REFERENCES

1. Stamey TA: *Pathogenesis and Treatment of Urinary Tract Infections*. Baltimore: Williams & Wilkins; 1980.

2. Brunner H, Weidner W, Schiefer HG: Studies on the role of *Ureaplasma urealyticum* and *Mycoplasma hominis* in prostatitis. *J Infect Dis* 1983, 147:807–813.

3. Schaeffer AJ, Wendel EF, Dunn JK, Grayhack JT: Prevalence and significance of prostatic inflammation. *J Urol* 1981, 125:215–219.

4. Kirby RS, Lowe D, Bultitude MI, Shuttleworth KED: Intra-prostatic urinary reflux: An aetiological factor in abacterial prostatitis. *Br J Urol* 1982, 54:729–731.

5. Schaeffer AJ, Chmiel JS, Grayhack JT: Natural history of prostatic inflammation [abstract]. *In Abstracts of the Annual Meeting of the American Urological Association*. 1985:207A.

6. Meares EM Jr: Prostatitis: A review. *Urol Clin North Am* 1975, 2:3–27.

7. Meares EM Jr: Prostatitis syndromes: New perspectives about old woes. *J Urol* 1980, 123:141–147.

8. Meares EM Jr Stamey TA: Bacteriologic localization patterns in bacterial prostatitis and urethritis. *Invest Urol* 1968, 5:492–518.

9. Meares EM Jr: Prostatitis and related disorders. *In* Walsh PC, Gittes RE, Perlmutter AD, Stamey TA (eds.): *Campbell's Urology*, 5th ed. Philadelphia: W.B. Saunders; 1986:868–887.

10. Stamey TA, Meares EM Jr, Winningham DG: Chronic bacterial prostatitis and the diffusion of drugs into prostatic fluid. *J Urol* 1970, 103:187–194.

11. Meares EM Jr: Prostatitis: Review of pharmacokinetics and therapy. *Rev Infect Dis* 1982, 4:475–483.

12. Wright AJ, Walker RC, Barrett DM: The fluoroquinolones and their appropriate use in treatment of genitourinary tract infections. *AUA Update Series* 1993, XII(7):49–56.

13. Meares EM Jr: Chronic bacterial prostatitis: Role of transurethral prostatectomy (TURP) in therapy. *In* Weidner W, Brunner H, Krause W, Rothauge CF (eds.): *Therapy of Prostatitis*. Munchen, Germany: W. Zuchsschwerdt Verlag; 1986:193–197.

14. Schwarz J: Mycotic prostatitis. *Urology* 1982, 19:1–5.

15. Bruce AW, Chadwick P, Willet WS, *et al.*: The role of chlamydiae in genitourinary disease. *J Urol* 1981, 126:625–629.

16. Thin RN, Simmons PD: Chronic bacterial and nonbacterial prostatitis. *Br J Urol* 1983, 55:513–518.

17. Shortliffe LMD, Elliott KM, Sellers RG, *et al.*: Measurement of chlamydial and ureaplasmal antibodies in serum and prostatic fluid of men with nonbacterial prostatitis [abstract]. *In Abstracts of Annual Meeting of American Urological Association*. 1985:276A.

18. Meares EM Jr: Acute and chronic prostatitis. *Infect Dis Clin North Am* 1987, 1:855–873.

19. Weidner W, Brunner H, Krause W: Quantitative culture of *Ureaplasma urealyticum* in patients with chronic prostatitis or prostatosis. *J Urol* 1980, 124:62–67.

20. Brock DJ, Grieco MH: Cryptococcal prostatitis in a patient with sarcoidosis: Response to 5-fluorocytosine. *J Urol* 1972, 107:1017–1021.

21. Lief M, Sarafarazi F: Prostatic cryptococcus in acquired immune deficiency syndrome. *Urology* 1986, 28:318–319.

22. O'Dea MJ, Hunting DB, Greene LF: Non-specific granulomatous prostatitis. *J Urol* 1977, 118:58–60.

23. Meares EM Jr: Prostatodynia: Clinical findings and rationale for treatment. *In* Weidner W, Brunner H, Krause W, Rothauge CF (eds.): *Therapy of Prostatitis*. Munchen, Germany: W. Zuchsschwerdt Verlag; 1986:207–212.

SELECTED BIBLIOGRAPHY

Cohen MS: Prostatic abscess. *In* Resnick MI, Kursh E (eds.): *Current Therapy in Genitourinary Surgery*, 2nd ed. Toronto: B.C. Decker; 1992:384–387.

Lim DJ, Schaeffer AJ: Prostatitis syndromes. *AUA Update Series* 1993, XII(1):1–8.

Meares EM Jr, Stamey TA: Bacteriologic localization patterns in bacterial prostatitis and urethritis. *Invest Urol* 1968, 5:492–518.

Meares EM Jr: Prostatitis. *Med Clin North Am* 1991, 75:405–424.

Schaeffer AJ, Wendel EF, Dunn JK, Grayhack JT: Prevalence and significance of prostatic inflammation. *J Urol* 1981, 125:215–219.

CHAPTER 5

Candiduria

Harry A. Gallis
Jack D. Sobel

EPIDEMIOLOGY

Trends in nosocomial *Candida* UTIs

Candida spp accounted for 7% of nosocomial infections in 1986–1989
Candida UTIs accounted for 9% of nosocomial UTIs, making them the 4th most common etiology
Overall, the frequency of *Candida* infections has increased by 200%–300% in the 1980s
90% of *Candida* UTIs are related to catheters or other instrumentation

UTI—urinary tract infection.

FIGURE 5-1 Trends in nosocomial *Candida* urinary tract infections. *Candida* infections have increased in frequency in all sites over the past 25 years. This increase is primarily due to the increased complexity of illness seen in hospitalized patients, such as immunocompromise and multiple trauma, as well as the increased use of broad-spectrum antibacterial agents [1–3].

Incidence of candiduria in hospitalized patients

1970s	Incidence increased from 1% to 9% of urinary tract infections
	One study noted incidence to be 11%
1980s	National Nosocomial Infections Surveillance = 9%
	Increased trend continues
1990s	Yeast species are found in < 1% of clean-voided specimens in healthy individuals

FIGURE 5-2 Incidence of candiduria in hospitalized patients. *Candida* species have risen to fourth among the causes of hospital-acquired urinary tract infections. The risk of further dissemination from the urinary tract has been studied in high-risk patients, but it may be as low as 1% overall [1,4,5].

Microbiology of candiduria

Candida albicans	> 50%
Torulopsis glabrata	≈ 25%
Candida tropicalis	5%–15%
Candida parapsilosis	5%–10%
Other *Candida* spp	5%–20%

FIGURE 5-3 Microbiology of candiduria. The percentage of individual species causing candiduria is approximated because many hospitals do not speciate non-*albicans* isolates from the urine. Non-*albicans Candida*, especially *C. glabrata*, is more commonly found in the urinary tract than in the oropharynx, esophagus, and vagina. Mixed infections with two or more *Candida* species are common in complicated urinary tract infections in catheterized patients.

Predisposing factors in candiduria

Previous/concurrent antibiotic therapy	90%
Bladder catheterization, other indwelling devices	85%
Less documented factors	
Female gender	
Obstruction of urinary tract	
Recent urologic surgery	
Renal transplantation	
Diabetes	
Corticosteroid therapy	
Coexistent bacteriuria	

FIGURE 5-4 Predisposing factors in candiduria. Numerous factors are thought to play a role in the genesis of candiduria. However, the presence of an indwelling urinary device and use of broad-spectrum antibiotics seem to play the largest part. Female gender, because of the vaginal reservoir of *Candida*, may also be a more significant risk factor [6,7].

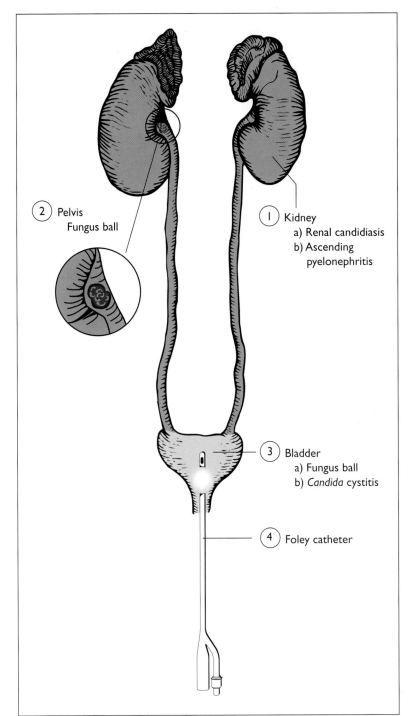

FIGURE 5-5 Anatomic sources of candiduria. The various *Candida* species that cause infection frequently are part of the normal flora of the gastrointestinal tract. Candiduria may reflect a renal, ureteric, bladder, or foreign body source. Most commonly, candiduria results from a lower urinary tract source.

(2) Pelvis
Fungus ball

(1) Kidney
a) Renal candidiasis
b) Ascending
pyelonephritis

(3) Bladder
a) Fungus ball
b) *Candida* cystitis

(4) Foley catheter

DIAGNOSIS

Diagnostic criteria in candiduria

$\geq 10^3$ organisms/mL
Pyuria
Symptoms
  May be absent
  Fever, dysuria, frequency, etc.

FIGURE 5-6 Diagnostic criteria in candiduria. In contrast to the situation with bacteriuria, standard criteria have yet to be developed for the interpretation of colony counts in urine specimens for candiduria. Hence, criteria vary among the various populations studied in the medical literature. No consensus exists, but most investigators consider $\geq 10^3$ organisms per mL of urine on at least two occasions as representing "significant" candiduria (*ie*, true infection, not contamination). Likewise, in contrast to bacteriuria, significant candiduria may be seen in the absence of pyuria (5–10 leukocytes/high-power field), especially in catheterized patients.

Diagnostic studies in *Candida* urinary tract infection

At least two positive cultures of $\geq 10^3$ organisms/mL of urine
  with same *Candida* spp
Exclude *Candida* vaginitis as cause of false-positive culture via
  contamination
Serologic tests not useful
Absence of pyuria does not rule out infection
Symptoms variable and depend on level of infection

FIGURE 5-7 Diagnostic studies in *Candida* urinary tract infection. Quantification of *Candida* species is not useful in differentiating colonization from infection or in identifying the site of infection. Similarly, the presence of pseudohyphae or mycelia may result from catheter colonization or from true tissue invasion.

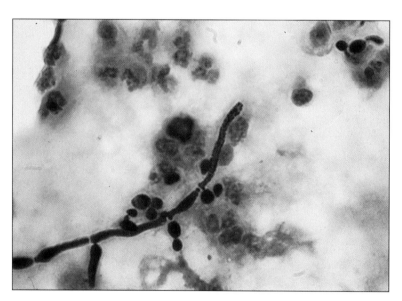

FIGURE 5-8 Pseudohyphae on Gram stain of urine sediment. Budding yeast and pseudohyphae are gram-positive and readily identified on Gram staining of urine. Pyuria is also present. (*Courtesy of* J.D. Sobel, MD.)

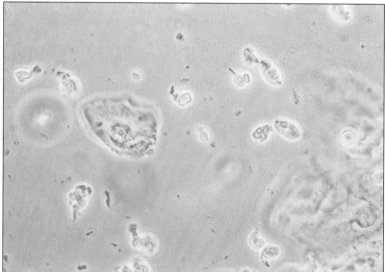

FIGURE 5-9 Unstained specimen of urine demonstrating multiple budding yeasts and rare uroepithelial cells. Absence of pseudohyphae suggests non-*albicans Candida* such as *C. glabrata*. (*Courtesy of* J.D. Sobel, MD.)

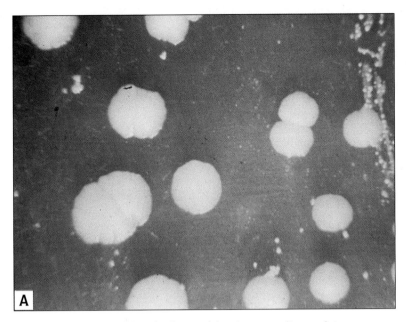

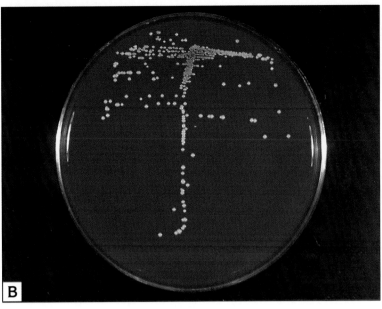

FIGURE 5-10 *Candida* colonies on blood agar culture plate.
A, *Candida* species initially produce small glistening white colonies on blood agar plates. Colonies may not be readily visible at 24 hours, but after 48 to 72 hours, the colonies may become more stellate and be more easily distinguished from bacterial colonies.

B, *Candida* colonies appear similar to *Staphylococcus*. To differentiate between them, Gram stain can be used to reveal the presence of budding cells, or wet mount examination will show fungal elements. (Panel 10A *courtesy of* J.D. Sobel, MD.)

PRINCIPLES OF MANAGEMENT

Clinical syndromes of *Candida* urinary tract infection

Asymptomatic candiduria
Candida cystourethritis
Ascending pyelonephritis
Hematogenous renal candidiasis
Fungus balls

FIGURE 5-11 Clinical syndromes of *Candida* urinary tract infection. The clinical syndromes caused by *Candida* infection of the urinary tract depend on the anatomic level of infection as well as the presence or absence of obstruction. The overwhelming majority of candiduria episodes originate from the lower urinary tract.

Distinguishing between upper and lower source of candiduria

Serologic tests of invasive candidiasis unreliable
Amphotericin B bladder washout/irrigation is only
    useful test
        Conventional testing requires 5-day irrigation
        48-hr or shorter duration irrigation may show similar
        clinical prediction
        Following irrigation, immediate recurrence of
        candiduria suggests upper tract disease
Presence of tubular casts containing yeasts and/or
    pseudohyphae indicative of renal involvement

FIGURE 5-12 Distinguishing between upper and lower source of candiduria. Localizing the site or source of candiduria forms the basis of treatment recommendations. Localization can be extremely difficult given the absence of reliable serologic tests of tissue invasion by *Candida*. Radiologic tests similarly have low sensitivity in determining the level of infection. At present, amphotericin B bladder washing is the only useful test, but its sensitivity and specificity have not been well documented. The presence of fungus balls or renal obstruction may suggest upper tract disease [8,9].

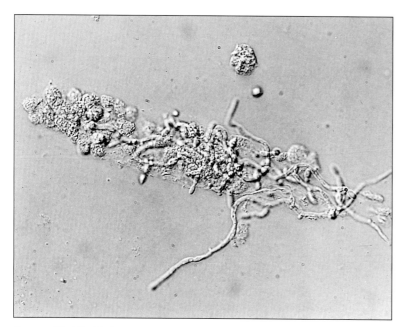

FIGURE 5-13 Light microscopy of renal tubular casts containing *Candida albicans* blastospores and mycelia, indicating renal parenchymal origin. When found on urine examination, this rare finding localizes infection to the kidney. (*Courtesy of* T. Walsh, MD.)

Treatment of candiduria: Factors to consider

Symptomatic vs asymptomatic
Catheter vs noncatheter
Suspected level of infection
Transplantation or other immunosuppression
Evidence of obstruction or upper tract disease
Urologic manipulation or surgery planned

FIGURE 5-14 Factors to consider in the treatment of candiduria. These factors should be taken into consideration in deciding whether antifungal therapy is indicated as well as in selecting the route, dose, and duration of antifungal agent.

Treatment of candiduria: Mechanical issues

Indwelling catheters are the single most common predisposing factor, so these should be dealt with first
Care must be taken to ensure that the patient can actually empty the bladder and that normal voiding mechanisms are reestablished following removal of catheter
Structural abnormalities and/or obstructions identified must be corrected or relieved immediately to prevent progression to urosepsis or relapse

FIGURE 5-15 Mechanical issues in the treatment of candiduria. In the presence of a foreign body in the urinary tract, such as a stent to relieve urinary obstruction, candiduria frequently persists despite putative adequate antifungal therapy until the foreign body is removed.

Treatment of candiduria: Lack of consensus

Analysis of treatment trials is confounded by:
Spontaneous recovery
Lack of diagnostic criteria
Lack of prospective randomization
Lack of ideal agent

FIGURE 5-16 Lack of consensus in the treatment of candiduria. Recommendations concerning treatment are confounded by the absence of any randomized, prospective, comparative studies. Therefore, the data presented in the literature are clouded by the variables listed in the figure. In various descriptive studies, as many as 50% of cases resolve simply with removal of urinary catheters; hence, all treatment trials must control for this variable.

CLINICAL SYNDROMES

Asymptomatic Candiduria

Asymptomatic candiduria: Definition

Two or more consecutive positive urine cultures for same
  Candida spp
At least 10^3 organisms/mL of urine
Absent local or systemic symptoms

FIGURE 5-17 Definition of asymptomatic candiduria. The overwhelming majority of candiduria episodes occur in asymptomatic
patients. In most patients, a second culture is negative, indicating
transient infection or contamination in obtaining the urine
specimen.

Clinical profile of patients with asymptomatic candiduria

> 80% have multiple predisposing features:
  Nosocomial
  Debilitated
  Diabetes
  Postoperative
  Elderly
  Antibiotic use (current or recent)
  Indwelling urinary catheters
  Intensive care unit setting

FIGURE 5-18 Clinical profile of patient with asymptomatic
candiduria. The majority of patients with candiduria are asymptomatic elderly, often debilitated patients. Hospital units in which
candiduria is most common include nursing homes and intensive
care units, including neonatal units.

Clinical implications of asymptomatic candiduria

Most asymptomatic episodes never result in symptoms
Usually resolve spontaneously
Rare complications:
  Symptomatic cystitis
  Fungus ball formation/obstruction
  Prostatic abscess
  Ascending infection with pyelonephritis and consequent
    candidemia

FIGURE 5-19 Clinical implications of asymptomatic candiduria.
Most patients are identified on routine urinalysis or on cultures
taken to assess the urinary tract in the presence of an indwelling
catheter. Therefore, candiduria usually produces no symptoms.

Risk factors for progression of asymptomatic candiduria

Manipulation of urinary tract
  Instrumentation
  Surgery
Obstruction/stasis
Other causes need to be defined

FIGURE 5-20 Risk factors for progression of asymptomatic
candiduria. The natural history of asymptomatic candiduria is
that most patients resolve spontaneously, especially with discon-
tinuation of the indwelling device. Thus, no therapy is indicated.
However, certain patients are at risk of progression to symptomatic disease, other genitourinary complications, and possibly
candidemia, particularly those who are catheterized, have foreign
bodies or other devices, develop obstructions, or are undergoing
operative procedures [10,11].

Candiduria as a source of candidemia

A rare occurrence (3%–10% of candidemias)
Usually associated with:
    Urologic procedures
    Obstruction/stasis
    Anatomic abnormalities
    Foreign bodies
A large multicenter observational study found positive blood
    cultures in only 1% of randomly selected patients with
    candiduria

FIGURE 5-21 Candiduria as a source of candidemia. Despite the
common occurrence of candiduria, ascending infection with
candidemia rarely occurs. Only 3% to 10% of candidemias result
from an ascending infection [10].

Effect of catheter removal on asymptomatic candiduria

Candiduria may resolve in up to 50% of patients following
    removal of indwelling catheter
In 20% of patients, candiduria may recur following an
    intervening negative culture

FIGURE 5-22 Effect of catheter removal on asymptomatic
candiduria. Candiduria frequently resolves on removal of
catheters. However, early recurrence of candiduria is not uncommon and, when caused by the same *Candida* species, implies
relapse from a persistent source within the urinary tract (*eg,*
prostate in men or upper tract parenchymal lesions or fungus
balls in both genders.) Therefore, in high risk patients, follow-up
for several weeks may be necessary.

Treatment of asymptomatic candiduria

Is treatment ever indicated?
    Some investigators claim...NEVER!
    Most asymptomatic patients with long-term indwelling
    catheters do NOT require therapy

FIGURE 5-23 Treatment of asymptomatic candiduria: Is treatment
ever indicated? Most patients with asymptomatic candiduria do
not require therapy. The recent availability of safe, effective tria-
zole agents to eliminate candiduria has revealed general ignorance
regarding when to treat candiduria. Select patient populations in
whom asymptomatic candiduria should be treated still require
definition.

Treatment of asymptomatic candiduria

Treatment is justified if*:
    Postrenal transplantation
    Neutropenic patients
    Before urologic surgery or manipulation

*Following second positive culture.

FIGURE 5-24 Indications in the treatment of asymptomatic
candiduria. Treatment may not be necessary in any but high-risk
patients. Patients with candiduria following renal and other solid-
organ transplantation, neutropenia, and prior to urologic surgery
or manipulation should be treated. Whether patients with asymptomatic diabetes or patients with urolithiasis and candiduria
warrant treatment is unknown [10].

Candida Cystourethritis

Clinical manifestations of *Candida* cystourethritis

Rare
May occur with or without urinary catheter
Symptoms (any combination)
  Urinary frequency
  Hematuria
  Dysuria

FIGURE 5-25 Clinical manifestations of *Candida* cystourethritis. Clinical features of *Candida* cystourethritis are indistinguishable from those of bacterial cystitis. Symptomatic bladder infections due to fungi are rare, especially given the frequency of superficial bladder infection in catheterized patients.

Urologic examination in *Candida* cystourethritis

Cystoscopy may show:
  Mucosal hyperemia
  Hemorrhagic ulceration
  Pseudomembranes that bleed easily when scraped
Cystoscopy is rarely indicated unless candiduria is persistent
  or obstruction is suspected

FIGURE 5-26 Urologic examination in *Candida* cystourethritis. Macroscopic findings include bladder mucosal hyperemia, ulceration (especially hemorrhagic ulceration), and thrushlike pseudomembranes.

Treatment issues in *Candida* cystourethritis

Treatment is always indicated
Remove or correct underlying factors
Route of therapy depends on presence of catheter
No catheter
  In ambulatory patients, oral (systemic) azole therapy
  In hospitalized patients or those unable to tolerate oral
    treatment, local therapy can be instituted through a newly
    inserted catheter using amphotericin B or systemic azole
    (intravenous fluconazole)
Catheter
  Local bladder irrigation with amphotericin B or
    systemic azole

FIGURE 5-27 Treatment issues in *Candida* cystourethritis. Symptomatic *Candida* cystourethritis usually responds rapidly to local or systemic antifungal therapy, particularly because infection is superficial and deep tissue invasion is unusual. Persistent candiduria may indicate a rare fungus ball in the bladder or upper tract *Candida* infection.

Treatment of noncatheter-related symptomatic *Candida* cystourethritis: Systemic therapy

1. Oral fluconazole (200 mg/day × 7 days)
2. Ketoconazole or itraconazole—less effective due to low
   urinary drug concentrations
3. Oral flucytosine—effective but less experience and
   more toxicity
4. Intravenous amphotericin B (0.3 mg/kg × single dose)
5. Conventional systemic intravenous amphotericin B
   (5–7 days of 0.3 mg/kg/day)

FIGURE 5-28 Systemic therapy in the treatment of noncatheter-related *Candida* cystourethritis. Ketoconazole and itraconazole achieve poor urinary drug concentrations and produce unreliable therapeutic results. Oral fluconazole in limited studies appears highly effective, especially given the high concentrations of fluconazole achieved in urine [12].

Treatment of symptomatic Candida cystourethritis in presence of indwelling catheter

Change/replace catheter drainage system
Consider:
    Systemic therapy with amphotericin B or fluconazole
                or
    Local amphotericin B irrigation

FIGURE 5-29 Treatment of symptomatic *Candida* cystourethritis in the presence of an indwelling catheter. Symptomatic cystitis due to *Candida* species is rare in catheterized patients. Accordingly, comparative therapeutic data are not available. Local or systemic antimycotic regimens should be effective.

Topical amphotericin B irrigation/washout as therapy for candiduria
Usual course = 50 mg amphotericin B/L sterile water or D5W   through triple-lumen catheter × 7–14 days Shorter courses unproven and not subjected to rigorous analysis Efficacy rates as high as 90% with up to 40%–50% relapses Also useful for nephrostomy irrigation

FIGURE 5-30 Topical amphotericin B irrigation/washout as therapy for candiduria. A triple-lumen catheter can be used for the constant infusion of amphotericin B. This requires a catheter change and new catheter in patients who did not have this kind of tubing in place. The usual technique is to deliver the 1000 mL of solution evenly over a 24-hour period. If the infusate is diluted by urine flow 2:1, the minimum concentration in bladder urine should be 15 to 20 mg/L [13,14].

Ascending Pyelonephritis

Pathogenesis of ascending pyelonephritis

Rare—almost never occurs in anatomically normal
    genitourinary tract
Predisposing factors:
    Obstruction
    Stasis
    Diabetes
    Indwelling foreign bodies (*eg*, stents, stones, catheters)

FIGURE 5-31 Pathogenesis of ascending pyelonephritis. Ascending pyelonephritis is an exceedingly uncommon complication of candiduria and usually occurs in the setting of obstruction, foreign body, or diabetes. This usually connotes an infection of the renal calyceal system and may result in papillary necrosis resulting in further obstruction. This needs to be distinguished from hematogenous pyelonephritis, which usually results in multiple renal cortical abscesses.

Signs and symptoms of ascending pyelonephritis	
Fever	Vomiting
Chills	Hematuria
Abdominal or flank pain	Tissue in urine

FIGURE 5-32 Signs and symptoms of ascending pyelonephritis. Clinical manifestations of ascending *Candida* pyelonephritis are similar to those of any bacterial parenchymal infection of the kidney. However, symptoms may not always be present, or they may be confused with other concurrent illnesses. Occasionally, upper urinary tract infection is silent, with formation of a fungus ball in the dilated pelvis or hydronephrosis; these patients present with candiduria only.

Complications of ascending *Candida* pyelonephritis
Renal abscess Perinephric abscess Gas formation (emphysematous pyelonephritis) Candidemia Sepsis/septic shock

FIGURE 5-33 Complications of ascending *Candida* pyelonephritis. Complications of ascending pyelonephritis may arise from persistent obstruction, leakage of urine around anastomotic sites following renal transplantation, or placement of percutaneous nephrostomy tubes. Emphysematous pyelonephritis can usually be diagnosed on a plain film of the abdomen and can also occur in infection due to the more common enteric gram-negative rods.

Radiologic evaluation in ascending pyelonephritis

Urography or ultrasound may show:
  Fungus balls in collecting system
  Papillary necrosis
  Obstruction due to fungus balls or papillary necrosis
  Gas in or around kidneys

FIGURE 5-34 Radiologic evaluation in ascending pyelonephritis. Renal ultrasound evidence for hydronephrosis may be an invaluable finding. A plain film of the abdomen will usually detect emphysematous pyelonephritis. A percutaneous nephrostogram may aid in the visualization of foreign material in the collecting system and the localization of obstruction. Intravenous urography is frequently contraindicated in patients with high-risk diabetes.

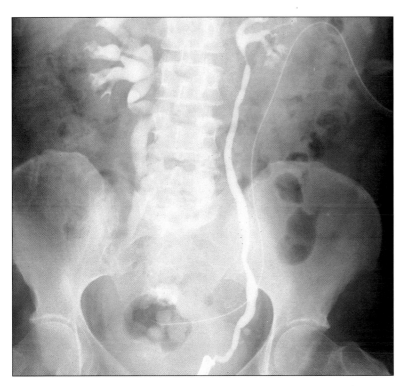

FIGURE 5-35 Retrograde pyelogram showing fungus ball with papillary necrosis. (*Courtesy of* J.D. Sobel, MD.)

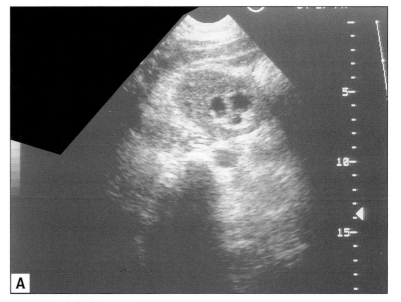

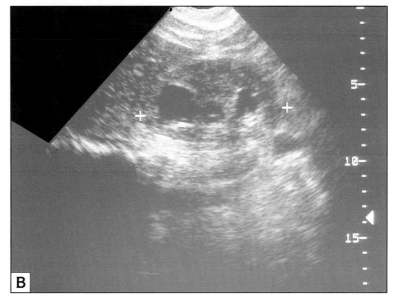

FIGURE 5-36 **A** and **B**, Ultrasound scans of ascending pyelonephritis showing fungus ball. (*Courtesy of* J.D. Sobel, MD.)

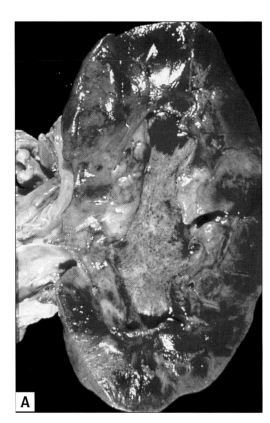

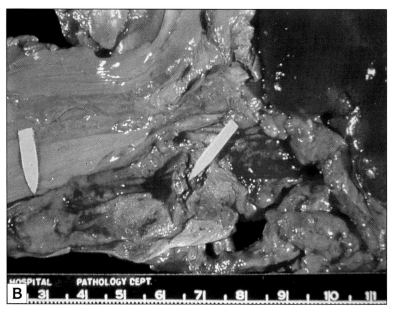

FIGURE 5-37 Gross pathology specimen of kidney showing fungus ball. **A,** A large, "fleshy" fungus ball is seen in the dilated pelvis of a hydronephrotic kidney. **B,** A large impacted fungus ball is seen in the dilated ureter (*arrows*). (*Courtesy of J.D. Sobel, MD.*)

Antifungal therapy for ascending pyelonephritis	
Amphotericin B	Previous "gold standard" for systemic and renal candidiasis
	Has never been subjected to rigorous analysis
	Depending on setting and patient, use 0.3–0.6 mg/kg/day
	If more prolonged therapy is required, oral fluconazole could be continued after initial therapy with amphotericin B
Fluconazole	Considered equivalent to amphotericin B
	Well-absorbed with high urinary excretion; low toxicity
	400 mg/day intravenous or oral

FIGURE 5-38 Antifungal therapy for ascending pyelonephritis. Treatment of ascending pyelonephritis requires systemic therapy with agents that achieve adequate levels in renal tissue and urine, such as amphotericin B and fluconazole. The other azole drugs, itraconazole and ketoconazole, are not excreted in the urine in sufficient quantity to be predictable. Flucytosine, although having excellent absorption and renal distribution, is limited by its toxicities and relatively narrow spectrum of activity [8,11,15].

Adjunctive treatment of upper urinary tract disease

Systemic therapy only effective after obstruction or fungus ball is removed
Surgical management issues:
    Ureteric stent placement for relief of obstruction
    Nephrostomy tube drainage
    Surgical removal of fungus balls/debris
Role of amphotericin B or fluconazole for irrigation of nephrostomy tubes
    With relatively resistant fungal pathogens such as *Candida glabrata, C. lusitaniae,*
      or *Aspergillus,* local delivery of amphotericin B may be contemplated

FIGURE 5-39 Adjunctive treatment of upper urinary tract disease. Because fluconazole achieves excellent urine concentrations after oral or intravenous administration, irrigation should seldom be contemplated, except perhaps in the setting of renal insufficiency.

Management of upper tract disease in advanced renal failure

Common clinical problem, especially in patients with nephrolithiasis, diabetes
    mellitus, other obstructive uropathy
Implies poor urinary concentrations of amphotericin B and fluconazole
    Emphasizes need for local therapeutic measures such as direct irrigation
    Tubes should be placed to achieve distribution of drug to the upper and
      lower genitourinary tract
Nephrostomy may be lifesaving

FIGURE 5-40 Management of upper tract disease in advanced renal failure and obstructive uropathy. In patients with a history of renal insufficiency with or without obstructive uropathy, achievement of renal tissue and cidal urinary levels may be difficult and unpredictable. Candiduria complicating nephrolithiasis or other forms of obstructive uropathy may place the renal collecting system at great risk.

Renal Candidiasis

Renal candidiasis (hematogenous pyelonephritis)

Metastatic infection due to hematogenous seeding of kidneys
    secondary to candidemia (kidneys may or may not be primary
    source)
More common than ascending pyelonephritis but may be clinically silent
True incidence unknown, but kidney is commonest systemic
    target organ/site in candidemia
Pathology shows multiple cortical abscesses that generally
    cannot be visualized in genitourinary imaging studies

FIGURE 5-41 Renal candidiasis (hematogenous pyelonephritis). Hematogenous pyelonephritis may occur secondary to candidemia from any source, including intravenous catheters, wound infections, and most commonly, neutropenic patients. The rich blood supply of the kidney together with the unique tropism of the *Candida* organism for glomerular epithelial cells results in the kidney's being the most common target site for metastatic infection.

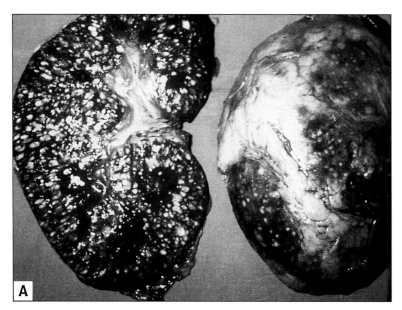

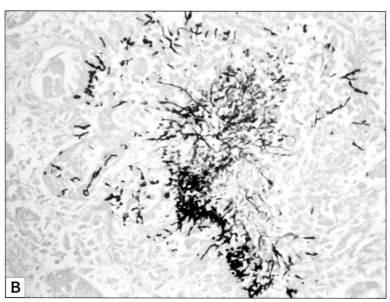

FIGURE 5-42 Pathology and histopathology specimens in renal candidiasis (hematogenous pyelonephritis). **A,** Gross pathology specimen of kidneys show multiple microabcesses scattered throughout the renal parenchyma. **B,** On histologic examination, microabscesses in the renal parenchyma with numerous hyphae are visible. (Gomori methenamine stain; original magnification, × 150.) (*Courtesy of* J.D. Sobel, MD.)

Clinical manifestations of renal candidiasis

1. Candiduria
2. Most patients have no symptoms referable to the kidney, presenting only with manifestations of candidemia
3. Fever may be only clinical manifestation
4. Progressive renal deterioration/impairment may occur
5. Rarely pain and hematuria

FIGURE 5-43 Clinical manifestations of renal candidiasis. Clinical manifestations of hematogenous candidiasis may be negligible or may be part of a syndrome of sepsis. Unfortunately, manifestations are subtle and nonspecific, resulting in a delay in diagnosis.

Diagnosis of hematogenous renal candidiasis

No reliable tests to detect renal invasion:
1. Serologic tests unreliable
2. Quantitative *Candida* antigen detection and polymerase chain reaction in the future
3. Rarely, renal tubular casts containing pseudohyphae may be present in urine
4. Candidemia frequently absent when candiduria discovered and renal candidiasis suspected

FIGURE 5-44 Diagnosis of hematogenous renal candidiasis. Diagnosis of hematogenous renal candidiasis is problematic because candidemia may be transient. The diagnosis is rarely confirmed, because of the absence of specific tests of tissue invasion. Radiologic studies are usually negative. Although deterioration in renal function frequently occurs, other causes of renal insufficiency often coexist.

FIGURE 5-45 Treatment of renal candidiasis. Management must be directed at the source, such as removal of intravenous catheters. Antifungal combination therapy with flucytosine is not specifically indicated. Renal function must be monitored.

Treatment of renal candidiasis

Identical to treatment of systemic candidiasis
Current recommendations:
1. Intravenous amphotericin B, 0.6–0.7 mg/kg/day
2. Intravenous fluconazole, 400–800 mg/day × 14 days (minimum)

OTHER FUNGAL ETIOLOGIES

Other fungal etiologies involving the genitourinary tract			
	Prostate	**Bladder**	**Kidney**
Blastomycosis	++	+	+
Histoplasmosis	++	+	++
Coccidioidomycosis	+	+	++
Aspergillosis	+	+	+++
Cryptococcosis	+++	+	+++
Candidiasis	+++	++++	++++

+—rare; ++++—common.

FIGURE 5-46 Other fungal etiologies involving the genitourinary tract. Numerous invasive mycoses may involve the urinary tract, inducing clinical syndromes depending on the site of infection. As indicated in the table, *Candida* species are by far the commonest fungi responsible for urinary tract infections. Prostatic infection may be symptomatic or serve as an asymptomatic reservoir for later reactivation.

REFERENCES

1. Schaberg DR, Culver DH, Gaynes RP: Major trends in the microbial etiology of nosocomial infection. *Am J Med* 1991, 91(suppl 3B):72S–75S.

2. Weber DJ, Rutala W, Samsa WA, *et al.*: Relative frequency of nosocomial pathogens at a university hospital during the decade 1980–1989. *Am J Infect Control* 1992, 20:192–197.

3. Stamm WE: Catheter-associated urinary tract infection: Epidemiology, pathogenesis, and prevention. *Am J Med* 1991, 91(suppl 3B):65S–71S.

4. Wise GJ, Goldberg P, Kozinn PJ: Genitourinary candidiasis: Diagnosis and treatment. *J Urol* 1976, 116:778–789.

5. Hamory BH, Wenzel RP: Hospital-associated candiduria: Predisposing factors and review of the literature. *J Urol* 1978, 120:444–448.

6. Gallis H, Vazquez J, Kauffman C, *et al.*: A prospective multicenter surveillance study of funguria in hospitalized patients [abstract 328]. Presented at the 33rd Meeting of the Infectious Diseases Society of America, San Francisco, 1995.

7. Fisher JF, Chew WH, Shadomy S, *et al.*: Urinary tract infections due to *Candida albicans. Rev Infect Dis* 1982, 4:1107–1118.

8. Hsu CCS, Ukleja B: Clearance of *Candida* colonizing the urinary bladder by a two-day amphotericin B irrigation. *Infection* 1990, 18:280–282.

9. Argyle C, Schumann GB, Genack L, Gregory M: Identification of fungal casts in a patient with renal candidiasis. *Hum Pathol* 1984, 15:480–481.

10. Ang BSP, Telenti A, King B, *et al.*: Candidemia from a urinary tract source: Microbiological aspects and clinical significance. *Clin Infect Dis* 1993, 17:662–666.

11. Wong-Beringer A, Jacobs RA, Guglielmo BJ: Treatment of funguria. *JAMA* 1992, 267:2780–2785.

12. Fisher JF, Hicks BC, Dipiro JT, *et al.*: Efficacy of a single intravenous dose of amphotericin B in urinary tract infections caused by *Candida* [letter]. *J Infect Dis* 1987, 156:685–687.

13. Sanford JP: The enigma of candiduria: Evolution of bladder irrigation with amphotericin B for management—From anecdote to dogma and a lesson from Machiavelli. *Clin Infect Dis* 1993, 16:145–147.

14. Gubbins PO, Piscitelli SC, Danziger LH: *Candida* urinary tract infections: A comprehensive review of their diagnosis and management. *Pharmacotherapy* 1993, 13:110–127.

15. Fisher JF, Newman CL, Sobel JD: Yeast in the urine: Solutions for a budding problem. *Clin Infect Dis* 1995, 20:183–189.

SELECTED BIBLIOGRAPHY

Fisher JF, Chew WH, Shadomy S, *et al.*: Urinary tract infections due to *Candida albicans. Rev Infect Dis* 1982, 4:1107–1118.

Gubbins PO, Piscitelli SC, Danziger LH: *Candida* urinary tract infections: A comprehensive review of their diagnosis and management. *Pharmacol Ther* 1993, 13:110–127.

Irby PB, Stoller MI, McAninch JW: Fungal bezoars of the upper urinary tract. *J Urol* 1990, 143:447–451.

Wong-Beringer A, Jacobs RA, Guglielmo BJ: Treatment of funguria. *JAMA* 1992, 267:2780–2785.

CHAPTER 6

Catheter-Associated Urinary Tract Infections

J. Curtis Nickel

URINARY CATHETERS

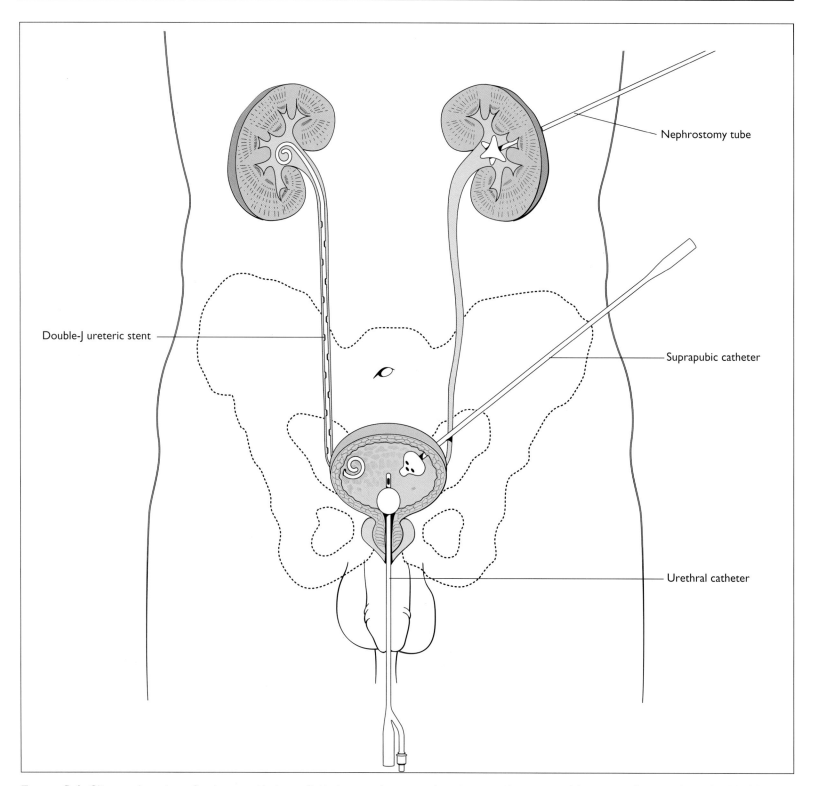

FIGURE 6-1 Sites and routes of urinary catheters. Catheters and stents are used to drain the bladder and kidneys. Catheters may be inserted into the bladder via the urethra or the percutaneous suprapubic route. The kidney can be drained with a percutaneous nephrostomy catheter or with a ureteric stent into the bladder. Approximately 15% of patients admitted to an acute care hospital will have some form of urinary catheter inserted during their hospital stay.

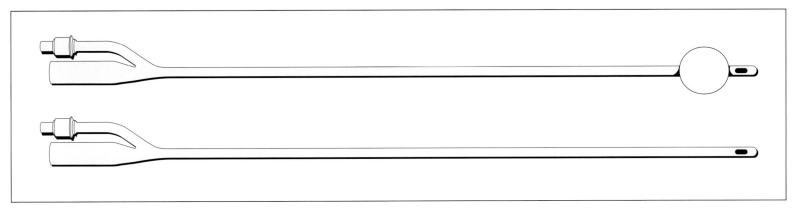

FIGURE 6-2 Foley catheter, inflated and deflated. The Foley catheter employs a unique proximal balloon at the tip of the catheter to anchor the device in the bladder. The balloon is inflated via a port at the proximal end of the catheter. The Foley catheter is the most common type of catheter used to drain the bladder.

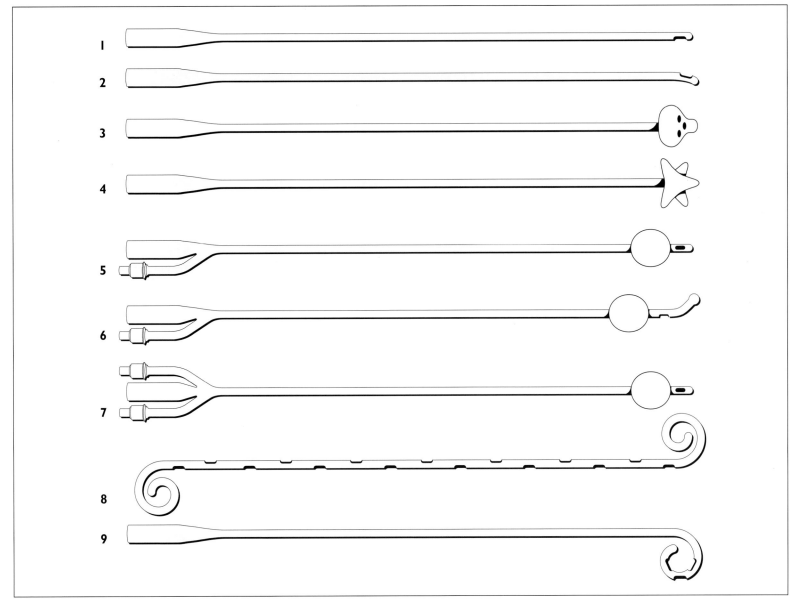

FIGURE 6-3 Types of urinary catheters. Different catheters are used for different reasons: (*1*) Simple urethral catheter—used for in- and out-catheterizations of the bladder. (*2*) Open-ended (whistle-tip) catheter—used to irrigate out bladder clots. (*3*) Mushroom or de Pezzer catheter—used for suprapubic or nephrostomy drainage. (*4*) Wing-tip or Malecot catheter—used for suprapubic or nephrostomy drainage. (*5*) Foley catheter with inflated retention balloon—used for urethral drainage of bladder. (*6*) Foley catheter with coudé tip—used as urethral catheter when difficulty negotiating a prostatic urethra is encountered or anticipated. (*7*) Three-way catheter—used for bladder irrigation. (*8*) Double-J catheter (stent)—used for indwelling ureteral drainage. (*9*) Single-J catheter—used for drainage of ureter and/or renal pelvis.

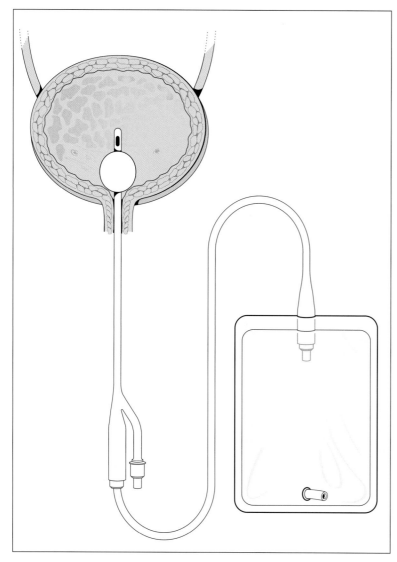

Uses of bladder catheters

Temporary or permanent relief of anatomic/physiologic
   urinary obstruction
Facilitates surgical repair of urethra, bladder, ureter, prostate
Provides dry environment for comatose or incontinent patients
Accurate measurement of urine output in severely ill patients

FIGURE 6-5 Use of bladder catheters. Catheters and stents are widely used in medical practice to relieve temporary anatomic or physiologic urinary obstruction, facilitate surgical repair of the urethral structures, provide a dry environment for comatose or incontinent patients, and permit accurate measurement of urine output in severely ill patients.

FIGURE 6-4 Closed urinary catheter system. Introduction of the closed urinary drainage system has been the most important technologic advance in the development of urinary drainage systems. The rate and frequency of acquired catheter-associated bacteriuria decreased significantly when these systems were universally employed. Although these systems have been modified many times over the past two decades, it is not entirely clear whether any of these modifications have subsequently reduced the infection rate from that attained with the original closed system.

Infection

↓

Excess morbidity
+
Three times increase in cost
+
Increased mortality

A

B. Hazards of urinary catheters

Infection
  Urethritis
  Urine infection (cystitis, pyelonephritis)
  Prostatitis, epididymitis (men)
  Sepsis
Urethral damage (erosion, strictures)
Expense
Mortality

FIGURE 6-6 Hazards of urinary catheters. **A** and **B**, Unfortunately, the indwelling catheter represents a definite hazard to the very patients it is designed to protect. It is associated with a significant excess morbidity (especially infection), high cost, and nearly threefold increase in mortality among hospitalized patients [1].

EPIDEMIOLOGY

Risk factors for acquired catheter-associated bacteriuria
Disconnection of catheter tubing junction
Improper catheter technique (insertion, drainage, care)
Duration of catheterization
Female sex
Elderly age
Debilitated status
Diabetes mellitus
Abnormal serum creatinine
Antimicrobial therapy

FIGURE 6-7 Risk factors for acquired catheter-associated bacteriuria. The risks of acquisition of catheter-associated bacteriuria is related to the sex and age of the patient as well as to the type and severity of underlying disease. Critical factors that can be altered are the duration of catheterization, techniques of catheter insertion and care (closed dependent drainage), and the possible use of systemic antimicrobial therapy in short-term catheterization and misuse in long-term catheterization [2].

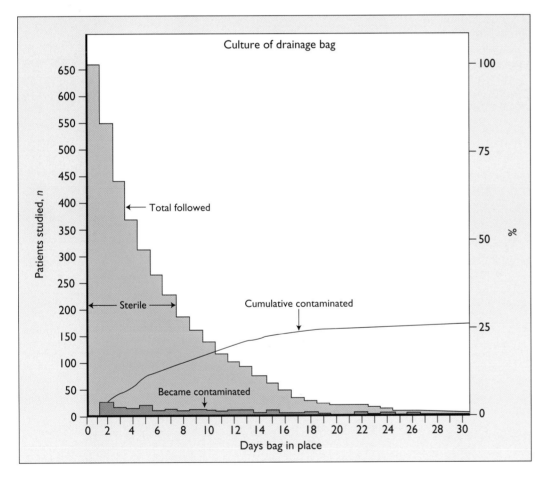

FIGURE 6-8 Increasing rates of infection with increased duration of catheterization. Infections in patients with indwelling catheters occur at a rate of 5% to 10% per day of catheterization, and at 30 days, almost 100% of catheterized patients will have bacteriuria. This graph shows the results of daily culture of urine from the catheter attached to a sterile closed urinary drainage bag in 662 consecutive patients studied in a general hospital. (*From* Kunin and McCormack [3]; with permission.)

PATHOGENESIS AND ETIOLOGY

A. Routes of infection in catheter-associated urinary tract infections

During introduction of catheter
Intraluminal route
Periurethral route

FIGURE 6-9 Routes of infection in catheter-associated urinary tract infection. **A** and **B**, Bacteria gain entrance to the bladder and urinary tract by few routes. Large numbers may be introduced when the catheter is passed (*1*), especially if improper aseptic technique is used. Later, bacteria may enter through the lumen of the catheter (intraluminal, *2*) or alongside an indwelling catheter in the periurethral space (extraluminal, *3*). Once the catheter is inserted, bacteria enter the drainage system from a contaminated drainage spout (*2a*), then pass through the drainage bag, which acts as a bacterial reservoir, and quickly ascend along the inside surface of the catheter itself. Ascent via this route can be accelerated if the catheter drainage tube junction is disconnected (*2b*). If proper closed drainage is maintained, the periurethral route, although slower, becomes the predominant route of infection [4].

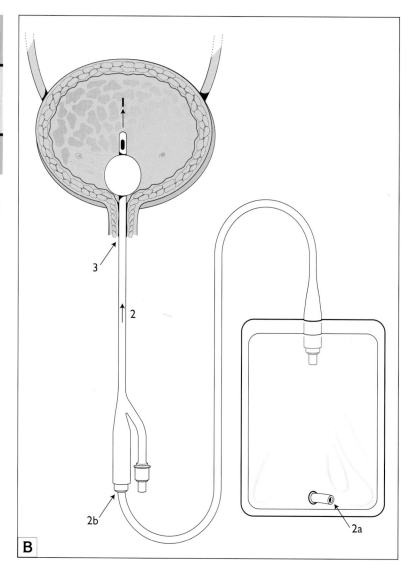

B

Bacterial virulence factors specific to catheter-associated urinary tract infections

Bacterial adherence to catheter material
Bacterial adherence to urethral and uriepithelial surfaces
Formation of bacterial biofilm

FIGURE 6-10 Bacterial virulence factors specific to catheter-associated urinary tract infection. Urinary tract infections occurring in patients who are not catheterized are related to the ability of the organism to adhere to the urothelium. In the pathogenesis of catheter-associated bacteriuria, the bacteria must be able to adhere to the catheter surface, whether intraluminal or extraluminal. Bacteria that can form aggregates or bacterial biofilms are able to spread along the catheter surfaces. Bacterial adherence is also important in colonization of the urethral meatus, which precedes the periurethral route of bacterial ascent into the bladder. Finally, bacterial adherence to the urothelium is the major factor that converts an asymptomatic bacteriuria to a symptomatic cystitis.

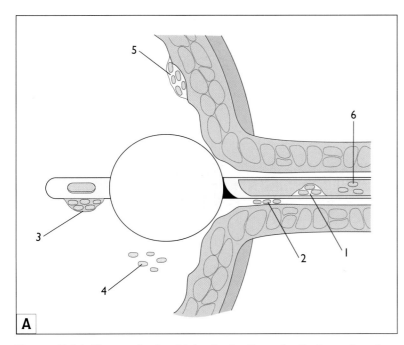

B. Types of microbial colonization of catheters

1. Coherent bacterial biofilm ascends the intraluminal surface of catheter against urine flow
2. Slower, thinner biofilm ascends extraluminal surface of catheter along periurethral mucus
3. Thicker or macroscopic bacterial biofilm or aggregate attach to intravesicular portion of catheter
4. Planktonic bacteria in nonbiofilm form (free-floating) present in urine between catheter and bladder surfaces
5. Bacteria adhere to bladder wall, which causes symptomatic bladder-associated infection
6. Planktonic bacteria wash down the catheter from bladder and can incorporate other bacterial populations 1–5

FIGURE 6-11 Types of microbial colonization of catheters. **A** and **B**, A number of distinct but interrelated microbial populations can be associated with catheter-associated urinary tract infections. Some of these populations are bacterial aggregates or biofilms that adhere to the catheter surface or bladder wall. The development of the infection appears to involve the intraluminal migration of this bacterial biofilm from an infected drainage spout, or, alternatively, ascent of the biofilm along the extraluminal surface of the catheter in the periurethral space from the urethral meatus. The existence of the first four populations listed in the figure results in catheter-associated bacteriuria, but at this point cystitis or symptomatic urinary tract infection has not occurred. Bacteria must become adherent to the bladder wall (as in population *5*) before symptomatic bladder-associated infection occurs. The planktonic bacteria being washed down the catheter from the bladder can incorporate any or all of the bacteria in populations *1* to *5* [5].

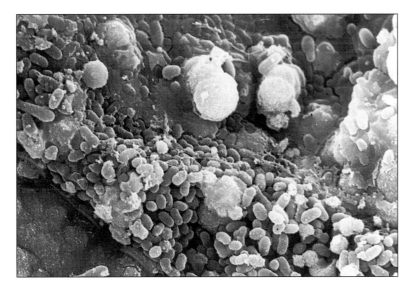

FIGURE 6-12 Scanning electron micrograph of the luminal surface of a colonized catheter. Bacterial cells within coherent biofilms are almost completely buried in a condensed slimelike glycocalyx. In some areas, the glycocalyx has been lost during preparation, disclosing the bacterial nature of the thick biofilm (*lower section*) as well as the surface of the catheter (*lower left corner*). (*From* Nickel *et al.* [6]; with permission.)

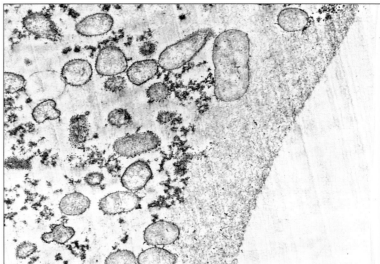

FIGURE 6-13 Transmission electron micrograph of a ruthenium red-stained antibody-stabilized preparation of the luminal surface of a pseudomonas biofilm. Antibody stabilization of the surface demonstrates the fibrous anionic matrix binding the bacterial cells together into the biofilm. Through a number of mechanisms, this matrix protects the bacteria within the biofilm from antibiotics, even though individual bacteria remain susceptible [7]. (*From* Nickel *et al.* [8]; with permission.)

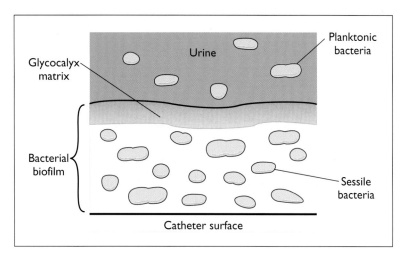

FIGURE 6-14 Diagram of the bacterial biofilm. Sessile bacteria are enmeshed in an exopolysaccharide glycocalyx matrix, which provides both adhesion to the catheter surface and protects from substances and antibiotics that would kill individual bacteria (planktonic bacteria) in the urine itself [9].

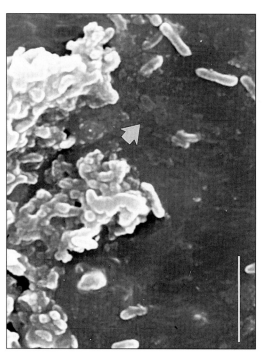

FIGURE 6-15 Scanning electron micrograph of an advancing front of a bacterial biofilm. Dehydrated glycocalyx matrix slime has condensed onto the bacterial aggregates. Both progressive and saltatory movements of biofilm can be noted. The *arrow* indicates the direction of movement. (Bar=5 μm.) (*From* Nickel *et al.* [8]; with permission.)

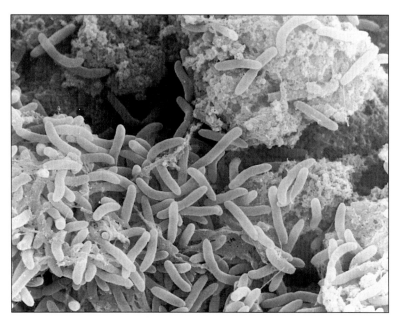

FIGURE 6-16 Scanning electron micrograph of an experimental bacterial biofilm ascending the luminal surface of a Foley catheter. The bacteria are seen advancing from the lower left, onto the catheter surface in the upper right. (*From* Nickel *et al.* [6]; with permission.)

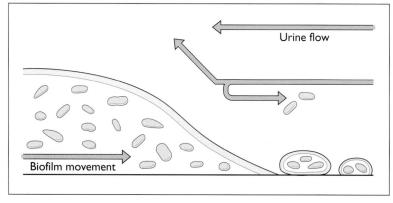

FIGURE 6-17 Diagram of an ascending bacterial biofilm demonstrating both progressive and saltatory movements. (*Adapted from* Nickel *et al.* [8].)

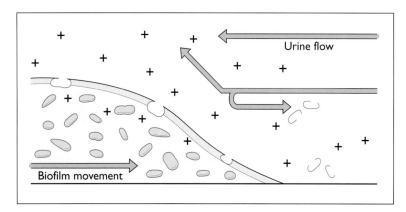

FIGURE 6-18 Effect of antibiotics on biofilm progression. Antibiotics, indicated by *plus signs*, significantly slow biofilm progress by precluding saltatory movement by killing unprotected planktonic bacteria and either stopping or reducing the metabolic activity of bacteria at the biofilm surface. (*Adapted from* Nickel *et al.* [8].)

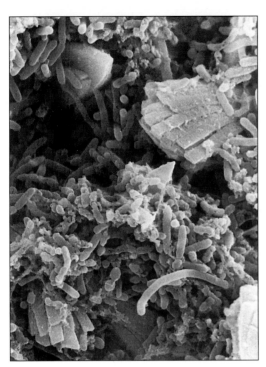

FIGURE 6-19
Scanning electron micrograph of the surface of an encrusted catheter showing rod-shaped and coccoid bacteria among the enveloping exopolysaccharide glycocalyx and uromucoid slime. Discrete crystals are noted within this coherent biofilm. The association of bacteria, slime, and crystals leads to eventual obstruction of the catheter or stent. (*From* Nickel et al. [10]; with permission.)

Microbiology of catheter-associated urinary tract infections

Escherichia coli
Enterococcus faecalis
Pseudomonas aeruginosa
Klebsiella spp
Enterobacter spp
Serratia spp
Proteus spp
Staphylococcus spp
Candida spp

FIGURE 6-20 Microbiology of catheter-associated urinary tract infection. Infections associated with catheterization are often mixed. *Escherichia coli* is common but so are other gram-negative bacilli that are rarer in primary infection. Gram-positive organisms, including *Enterococcus* and *Staphylococcus*, are also more common in catheter-associated urinary tract infections. Various *Candida* species and other related yeasts can be important in diabetic, debilitated, and/or patients receiving wide-spectrum antibiotics. In patients who are not receiving antibacterial medication, *E. coli* and *Enterococcus* and *Proteus* species appear to be implicated in most cases of bacteriuria, whereas in patients receiving prophylactic antibiotic therapy, *Pseudomonas*, *Candida*, *Serratia*, and others cause most infections.

CLINICAL ASPECTS OF CATHETER-ASSOCIATED URINARY TRACT INFECTIONS

Clinical manifestations of catheter-associated cystitis

Asymptomatic bacteriuria
Symptomatic cystitis
Bacteremia/septicemia (urosepsis)

FIGURE 6-21 Clinical manifestations of catheter-associated urinary tract infections. Bacteriuria associated with an indwelling Foley catheter is usually asymptomatic. Bacteria colonize the catheter surface and are present in the thin film of urine between the catheter and bladder wall. If the bacteria are particularly virulent, the mucosal surface is damaged, or catheter flow is altered, bacteria adhere in small microcolonies or aggregates to the epithelial surface, and symptomatic cystitis subsequently occurs. If significant catheter trauma to the urethra or bladder occurs or if the catheter becomes blocked, bacteria can be forced into the bloodstream and bacteremia and possibly septicemia results. Most cases of bacteremia are secondary to ascending pyelonephritis.

Manifestations of symptomatic catheter-associated urinary tract infections

Local	Systemic
Suprapubic pain	Fever
Bladder spasm	Chills
Hematuria	Rigors
Urethral pain, discharge	Abdominal pain
	Sepsis

FIGURE 6-22 Manifestations of symptomatic catheter-associated urinary tract infection. If bacteria colonizing the catheter surface or the thin film of urine coating the bladder adhere to and then invade the bladder wall, symptomatic cystitis may occur. This results in primarily local symptoms of suprapubic pain, bladder spasms, and hematuria. If urine flow through the catheter is altered, *ie*, catheter blocks, or urine refluxes into the kidneys, bacteria can enter the bloodstream and bacteremia can occur. This can quickly progress to septicemia and even septic shock.

Complications of catheter-associated urinary tract infections

Cystitis	Infected bladder calculi
Urethritis	Pyelonephritis
Periurethral abscess	Bacteremia/septicemia
Prostatitis and prostatic abscess	Septic shock
	Death
Epididymitis	

FIGURE 6-23 Complications of catheter-associated urinary tract infections. The complications of an indwelling Foley catheter can include local problems such as symptomatic cystitis and urethritis, prostatitis, and prostatic abscess if bacteria reflux into the prostatic ducts, and acute epididymitis if bacteria reflux up the vas deferens. If following ascending infection, bacteria enter the bloodstream, bacteremia results and septicemia is a possibility. Urinary catheters are still the leading cause of mortality from gram-negative nosocomial septic shock.

Diagnosis of catheter-associated urinary tract infections

1. Bacteriuria 10^2–10^5 colony-forming units per mL (?)
2. Pyuria
3. Microscopic hematuria

FIGURE 6-24 Diagnosis of catheter-associated urinary tract infections. There is much controversy as to what level of bacteriuria should be considered significant. If the bacteriuria is asymptomatic, then it is not clinically significant and catheter-associated infection should not be diagnosed or treated. However, if symptoms do occur, then any level of bacteriuria > 10^2 colony-forming units per mL could be significant. Similarly, pyuria inevitably occurs in catheterized patients and is unhelpful in deciding whether to initiate therapy. Hematuria can occur with catheter trauma as well as from cystitis. The diagnosis of catheter-associated cystitis has to be made on clinical grounds, including symptoms, physical findings, and determination of catheter-associated bacteriuria. The optimal way to obtain this urine specimen is by drawing a needle aspirate from the Foley catheter itself.

FIGURE 6-25 Procedure for obtaining urine specimens from catheterized patients. The most accurate way to obtain urine specimens for culture and antibiotic sensitivity testing is to insert a small-caliber needle into the shaft of the catheter and draw out the required aliquot of urine. This method avoids the inevitable contamination that results when urine from the drainage bag is cultured.

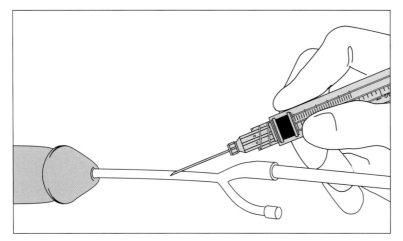

TREATMENT

Management of asymptomatic bacteriuria

1. Should rarely be treated
2. Indications for treatment:
   a. Prior to instrumentation of urinary tract
   b. Immunosuppressed patients
   c. Bacteriuria persisting after removal of catheter

FIGURE 6-26 Management of asymptomatic bacteriuria. Asymptomatic bacteriuria associated with indwelling catheters rarely needs to be treated. Treatment may be required when instrumentation of the urinary tract is contemplated or in some immunosuppressed patients (*eg*, kidney transplantation, chemotherapy). Bacteriuria persisting after the catheter has been removed, whether it is asymptomatic or not, probably should be treated with a short course of antibiotics.

FIGURE 6-27 Principles of treatment of catheter-associated urinary tract infection (UTI). Antibiotic therapy for catheter-associated UTIs should be based on culture results. However, broad-spectrum oral antibiotics for cystitis and wide-spectrum parenteral antibiotics for systemic infections should be started until the results of urine and/or blood cultures become available. Selection is facilitated by urine Gram stain. Ideally, the catheter should be removed (because it is a source of the pathogenic bacteria). If it is not needed, it should be left out. If catheter drainage is required, consideration should be given to intermittent catheterization. Once the infection has resolved and the catheter has been finally removed, test-of-cure cultures should be done. Catheter-associated infections are complicated UTIs, and the duration of therapy should reflect this fact.

Treatment of catheter-associated UTIs: Principles

1. Should be based on culture (urine and blood)
2. Catheter should ideally be removed during treatment or replaced if still indicated
3. These UTIs are complicated and should be treated from 7–14 days depending on severity
4. Cultures should be obtained after catheter is removed

UTI—urinary tract infection.

FIGURE 6-28 Selection of antibiotics in catheter-associated urinary tract infections. Asymptomatic bacteriuria should be treated rarely. Symptomatic cystitis is preferably treated with one of the broad-spectrum quinolones combined with catheter removal. Treatment of systemic catheter-associated urinary tract infections should include intravenous antibiotics that cover both gram-positive and gram-negative bacteria.

Selection of antibiotics in catheter-associated urinary tract infections

1. Asymptomatic bacteriuria
   Rarely if ever treated
2. Symptomatic cystitis
   Trimethoprim-sulfamethoxazole, quinolones, β-lactams
3. Systemic
   Ampicillin and gentamicin
   Third-generation cephalosporin
   Quinolones
   Extended-spectrum penicillin

FIGURE 6-29 Pitfalls of treatment of catheter-associated urinary tract infections (UTIs). The most frequent pitfall in managing catheters and bacteriuria is unnecessary treatment of asymptomatic patients. All patients with an indwelling catheter will develop bacteriuria eventually, and antibiotic treatment of bacteriuria without symptoms will select for more resistant organisms within the polymicrobial biofilm on the catheter surface. On the other hand, clinicians must learn to recognize when this bacteriuria becomes symptomatic, because then treatment is imperative. Serious sepsis results when the catheter becomes blocked, and this must be recognized and rectified. It is important to remove the offending catheter when treating the UTI and replace with a new catheter only if no other method of bladder drainage is available. Patients with catheter-associated UTIs whose catheter must remain in place tend to have recurrent episodes of symptomatic infections, and recognition of the associated factors is important to developing an individualized prevention program.

Treatment of catheter-associated UTIs: Pitfalls

1. Unnecessary treatment of asymptomatic bacteriuria
2. Unrecognized catheter-associated UTI
3. Failure to recognize blocked catheter
4. Failure to remove infected catheter
5. Attributing all fever in catheterized patient to UTI (exclude other causes)

UTI—urinary tract infection.

PREVENTION

Prevention of catheter-associated urinary tract infections: Principles

1. Avoid unnecessary catheterization
2. Sterile technique for insertion of catheter
3. Remove catheter as soon as possible
4. Closed drainage system
5. Ensure dependent drainage
6. Separation of infected catheterized patients

FIGURE 6-30 Principles of prevention of catheter-associated urinary tract infections. Infection control measures proven to prevent catheter-associated urinary tract infections include strict adherence to sterile techniques when initially inserting a catheter and maintenance of a closed urinary drainage system that flows downhill. Meticulous sterile care of the drainage spout, prevention of disruption to the catheter drainage tube junction, and excellent nursing care to prevent contamination between catheterized patients remain mandatory [11].

Prevention of catheter-associated urinary tract infections: Controversies

1. Care of urethral meatus
2. Antibiotic prophylaxis
3. Microbicidal agents in drainage bag and spout
4. Catheter material
5. Antimicrobial catheter coatings
6. Size of catheter
7. Catheter changes
8. High-volume urine output
9. Bacteriologic monitoring

FIGURE 6-31 Controversies of prevention of catheter-associated urinary tract infections. Excellent meatal care, including frequent cleaning and even antibiotic ointment, remains an important consideration in reducing the periurethral route of infection and maybe in preventing serious catheter-associated sequelae, such as urethral meatal stenosis. Theoretical findings and early clinical data suggest that prophylactic antibiotic coverage in short-term catheterization may reduce the incidence of catheter-associated infection and its serious sequelae. Antibiotic use in long-term chronic catheterization is not indicated and potentially harmful, because it selects out antibiotic-resistant organisms. Similarly, microbicidal agents introduced into the collecting bag or drainage spout reduce the rate of catheter-associated bacteriuria by the intraluminal route. Teflon- or silicone-coated catheters appear to reduce urethral irritation, and newer lubricous or hydrophilic catheters appear to have further improved urethral biocompatibility and perhaps even reduced infection rates. Incorporating antimicrobial substances into or onto the catheter itself theoretically may reduce bacterial adherence and subsequent infection. However, catheters impregnated with antibiotics have shown no real efficacy, but coating the catheter with silver or incorporating silver ions in a hydrophilic catheter coating has shown some promise. A catheter too large for the urethra will cause pressure necrosis of the urethra and subsequent urethritis. A catheter that is too small will block easier, increasing the chance of a resulting bacteremia. There is no rigid standard for the frequency of catheter changes, but some patients have more frequent blocks than others. A high-volume urine flow may keep the catheter patent for a longer period of time. Bacteriologic monitoring of urine to determine the bacteria and their antibiotic sensitivities would be useful if the patient did develop a symptomatic urinary tract infection, but generally this is not cost-effective and may lead to treatment of asymptomatic bacteriuria [12].

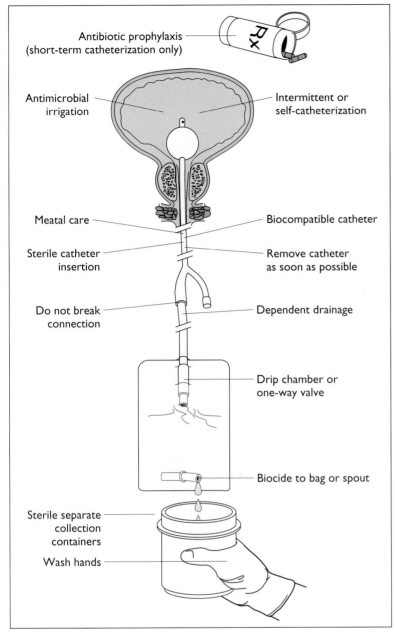

FIGURE 6-32 Infection control measures in closed drainage systems.

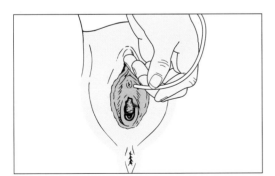

Prevention of catheter-associated urinary tract infections: Alternatives to chronic catheterization

Intermittent self-catheterization
Condom urinary drainage
Chronic suprapubic catheterization

FIGURE 6-33 Alternatives to chronic catheterization in the prevention of catheter-associated urinary tract infections. In patients who require urinary drainage, there are viable alternatives to a chronic indwelling Foley catheter. These alternatives include intermittent catheterization, condom urinary drainage, and suprapubic catheterization.

FIGURE 6-34 Intermittent self-catheterization. Patients who are unable to empty their bladder but have reasonable manual dexterity can be taught clean intermittent self-catheterization. Although episodes of urinary tract infections can occur, the long-term complications and sequelae can be drastically reduced when converting a patient from chronic indwelling Foley catheterization to intermittent catheterization.

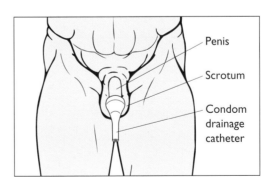

FIGURE 6-35 Condom urinary drainage. Patients, particularly men, who were catheterized primarily for incontinence can be managed with condom urinary drainage. This method significantly reduces the complications associated with a chronic indwelling catheter. Some patients with chronic urinary retention may require some form of bladder neck or urethral sphincter operation so that the bladder adequately drains without intubation.

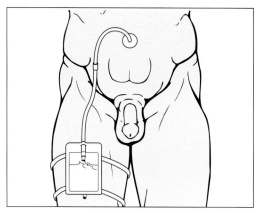

Figure 6-36 Chronic percutaneous suprapubic catheterization. In patients with urinary retention who must be managed with an indwelling catheter, percutaneous suprapubic catheterization avoids many of the serious complications and long-term sequelae of having a chronic catheter within the urethra. It is much more comfortable for the patient in the short-term, and in the long-term it reduces the rate of urethritis, urethral erosion, and, in men, prostatitis and epididymitis. The catheter does have to be changed routinely, and patients still develop chronic bacteriuria that occasionally can become symptomatic.

Future advances in the prevention and treatment of catheter-associated urinary tract infections

1. Biomaterial research
2. New antibiotics
3. Targeted antibiotic therapy
4. New advances in the treatment of cystitis

Figure 6-37 Future advances in the prevention and treatment of catheter-associated urinary tract infections. Biomaterials research is presently addressing factors that are implicated in catheter-associated urinary tract infections, including mucosal biocompatibility, reducing bacterial adherence and biofilm formation on the catheter surface, and even development of a bacteriostatic or bacteriocidal catheter surface. The development of hydrophilic and antibacterial catheter coatings may prove efficacious in reducing such adherence. It has been demonstrated that the quinolones appear to penetrate the bacterial biofilm better than penicillins or aminoglycosides. Further research will lead to new antibiotics that may be able to eradicate bacterial aggregates adherent to prosthetic devices such as catheters. Future studies will allow us to rationalize antibiotic therapy both to prevent and treat catheter-associated infection. Antibiotic prophylaxis in short-term catheterization may prove to be clinically acceptable. Selective gut decontamination may be the mechanism by which this type of antibiotic therapy for short-term catheterization may work. New advances in the treatment of cystitis, by increasing bladder defense mechanisms either immunologically or by improving the bladder surface mucin layer, are presently under study. The interaction of bacteria and the bladder surface may be one step amenable to future intervention. For now, the most effective way to reduce the incidence of catheter-associated infection is to avoid indwelling Foley catheterization if at all possible, or at least to reduce the length of time that the catheter remains in place.

REFERENCES

1. Platt R, Polk BF, Murdock B, Rosner B: Mortality associated with nosocomial urinary tract infection. *N Engl J Med* 1982, 307:637–642.

2. Garibaldi RA, Burke JP, Dickman ML, Smith CB: Factors predisposing bacteriuria during indwelling urethral catheterization. *N Engl J Med* 1974, 291:215–219.

3. Kunin CM, McCormack RC: Prevention of catheter-induced urinary tract infections by sterile closed drainage. *N Engl J Med* 1966, 274:1156–1161.

4. Thorton GF, Andriole VT: Bacteriuria during indwelling catheter drainage. *JAMA* 1970, 214:339–342.

5. Schaeffer AJ: Catheter-associated bacteriuria. *Urol Clin North Am* 1986, 13:735–747.

6. Nickel JC, Grant SK, Costerton JW: Catheter associated bacteriuria: An experimental study. *Urology* 1985, 26:369–375.

7. Nickel JC, Downey J, Costerton JW: An ultrastructural study of microbiological colonization of urinary catheters. *Urology* 1989, 34:284–291.

8. Nickel JC, Downey J, Costerton JW: Movement of *Pseudomonas aeruginosa* along catheter surfaces: A mechanism in the pathogenesis of catheter associated infection. *Urology* 1992, 39:93–98.

9. Nickel JC, Ruseska I, Wright JB, Costerton JW: Tobramycin resistance of *Pseudomonas aeruginosa* cells growing as a biofilm in urinary catheter material. *Antimicrob Agents Chemother* 1985, 27:619–624.

10. Nickel JC, Emtage J, Costerton JW: Ultrastructural microbial ecology of infection-induced urinary stones. *J Urol* 1985, 133:622–627.

11. Stamm WE: Guidelines for the prevention of catheter associated urinary tract infections. *Ann Intern Med* 1975, 82:386–390.

12. Nickel JC, Costerton JW: Bacterial biofilms and catheters: A key to understanding bacterial strategies in catheter-associated urinary tract infection. *Can J Infect Dis* 1992, 3:261–267.

SELECTED BIBLIOGRAPHY

Kunin CM: Care of the urinary catheter. *In Detection, Prevention and Management of Urinary Tract Infection.* Philadelphia, Lea & Febiger; 1987:245–297.

Nickel JC, Costerton JW: Bacterial biofilms and catheters: A key to understanding bacterial strategies in catheter-associated urinary tract infection. *Can J Infect Dis* 1992, 3:261–267.

Schaeffer AJ: Catheter associated bacteriuria. Urol Clin North Am 1986, 13:735–747.

Stamm WE: Catheter-associated urinary tract infections: Epidemiology, pathogenesis, and prevention. *Am J Med* 1991, 91(suppl 3B):65–71.

Stamm WE: Guidelines for the prevention of catheter associated urinary tract infections. *Ann Intern Med* 1975, 82:386–390.

CHAPTER 7

Infections of the Vulva

Elaine T. Kaye

NORMAL AND ABNORMAL ANATOMY

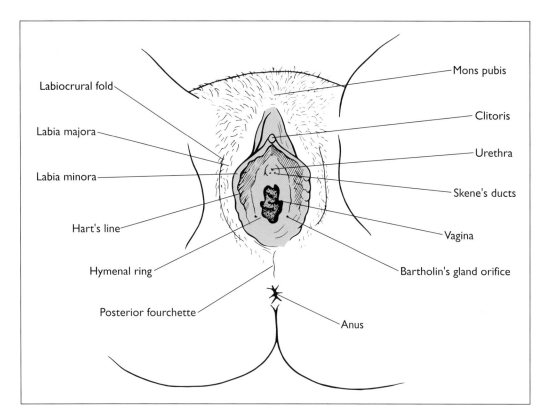

Labiocrural fold

Labia majora

Labia minora

Hart's line

Hymenal ring

Posterior fourchette

Mons pubis

Clitoris

Urethra

Skene's ducts

Vagina

Bartholin's gland orifice

Anus

FIGURE 7-1 Schematic depiction of the vulva. The vulva includes the labia majora, labia minora, clitoris, and vulvar vestibule. Its lateral borders are the labiocrural folds, and its central boundary is the hymen. The anterior and posterior boundaries are the mons pubis and anus, respectively.

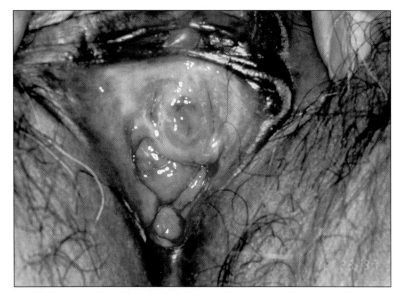

FIGURE 7-2 Aged vulva. The typical aged, parous vulva with laxity of all structures, including the vaginal orifice, is pictured. There is also subluxation of the vaginal wall and shrinkage of the labia minora with its smooth, glistening, and patchy erythematous lining. (*Courtesy of* S.C. Marinoff, MD, and M. Turner, MD, *from* American Academy of Dermatology [1], with permission.)

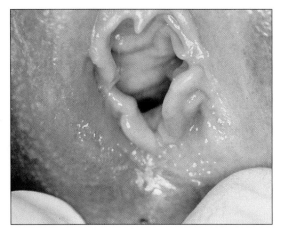

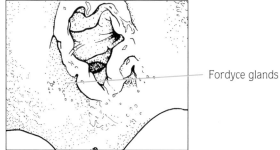

Fordyce glands

FIGURE 7-3 Fordyce glands. Fordyce glands are sebaceous glands that open directly onto the surface of the stratified epithelium, visible here as yellow papules. Orifices of minor vestibular glands are located at the base of the hymen. (*Courtesy of* M. Turner, MD; *from* American Academy of Dermatology [1], with permission.)

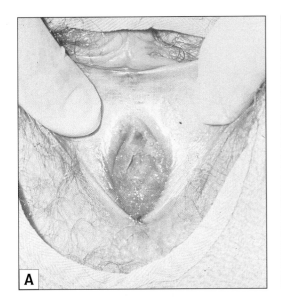

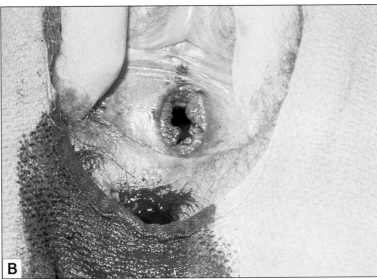

Figure 7-4 Imperforate hymen. The hymen is a thin membranous structure separating the vulvar vestibule from the vagina. The hymen demarcates the central boundary of the vulva. **A,** The congenital abnormality of the imperforate hymen. **B,** Surgical correction of the hymen, immediately postoperatively. The hymen is now patent. (*Courtesy of* M. Spence, MD.)

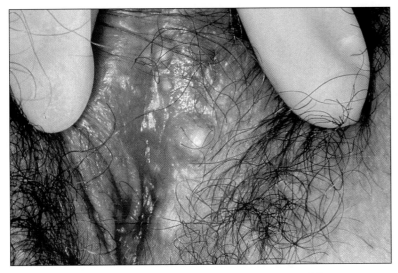

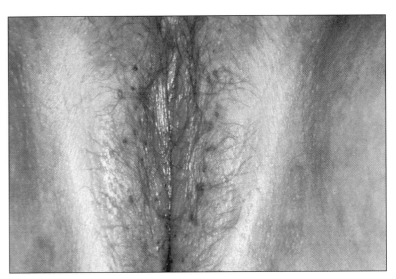

Figure 7-5 Epidermal inclusion cysts. These firm, white to yellowish, smooth papules and nodules occur most commonly on the labia majora. They are sometimes called *sebaceous cysts,* which is a misnomer because they actually result from obstructed hair follicles or epidermis displaced by trauma. They may become inflamed and occasionally become infected, requiring antibiotics and drainage. Recurrences of the cysts are likely unless the cyst lining is removed surgically. (*Courtesy of* M. Turner, MD; *from* American Academy of Dermatology [1]; with permission.)

Figure 7-6 Angiokeratoma. Angiokeratomas occur as single or multiple, 2- to 10-mm papules in shades of red or blue and may be smooth or warty. They are analogous to scrotal angiokeratomas (Fordyce). (*Courtesy of* M. Turner, MD; *from* American Academy of Dermatology [1], with permission.)

DIFFERENTIAL DIAGNOSIS OF INFECTION

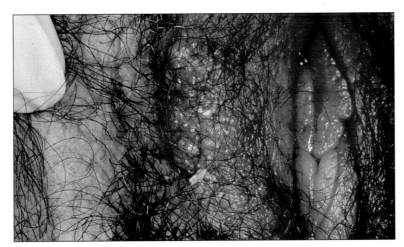

Figure 7-7 Lymphangioma. The clear grapelike groupings of small tense vesicles are caused by ectasia of lymphatic vessels that occurred several years after pelvic irradiation for lymphoma. The differential diagnosis includes herpes simplex, herpes zoster, and immunologic bullous disease such as pemphigus vulgaris. Lymphangioma usually can be distinguished from herpes by the scattered vesicles of long-standing and asymptomatic nature, as opposed to the painful, short-lived clusters of vesicles seen with herpes. The skin surrounding the vesicles of lymphangioma may also appear thickened or hyperkeratotic. (*Courtesy of* M. Turner, MD; *from* American Academy of Dermatology [1], with permission.)

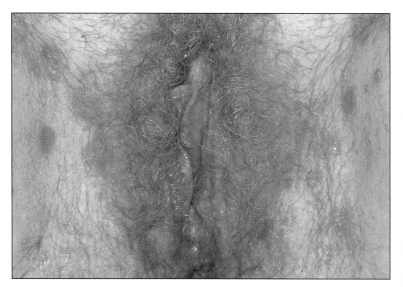

FIGURE 7-8 Psoriasis presenting as pink, well-demarcated plaques on the vulva. Psoriasis in the vulvar area or the intergluteal folds often lacks the typical micaceous scale seen elsewhere. Pruritus is the most common presenting symptom. The erythematous and scaly appearance may mimic candidal and dermatophyte infection. The presence of lesions in other typical areas of involvement, such as the elbows, knees, scalp, and umbilicus can help establish the diagnosis of psoriasis. (*Courtesy of* L. Edwards, MD.)

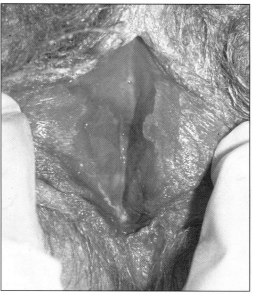

FIGURE 7-9 Contact dermatitis caused by 5-fluorouracil. Contact dermatitis is a type of eczematous dermatitis in reaction to an irritant or allergen. It presents with erythema and edema and, in more severe cases, with desquamation as seen here. The differential diagnosis includes atopic dermatitis, psoriasis, as well as fungal and bacterial skin infection. Because the findings on clinical examination may be nonspecific, the diagnosis often depends on a suggestive history. A thorough history is essential in identifying the offending agent, which may include a fragrance, preservative, or other chemical in products used by patients *or* their sexual partners. If the allergen cannot be identified and the dermatitis is recurrent, patch testing of common allergens may be helpful. (*Courtesy of* L. Edwards, MD.)

Allergens in implicated vulvar contact dermatitis	
Substance	**Example of offending agent**
Medications	
Anesthetics	Lidocaine
Antibiotics	—
Anticandidals	Azoles
Antiseptics	Povidine-iodine
Corticosteroids	—
Spermicides	—
Additives to personal hygiene products, cosmetics, medications	
Preservatives	Parabens
Fragrances	—
Emollients	—
Materials	
Panty liners, sanitary napkins	Formaldehyde
Condoms, diaphragms, examination gloves	Latex
Body fluids	Semen, saliva
Snaps, buckles, pins	Nickel
Clothing	Dyes
Nail polish	Toluene
Poison ivy, oak, and sumac	—

FIGURE 7-10 Allergens implicated in vulvar contact dermatitis. (*Adapted from* Lynch and Edwards [2].)

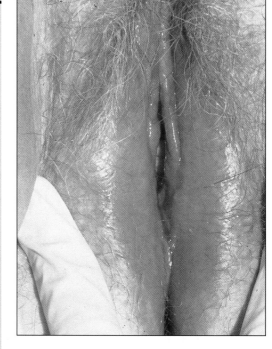

FIGURE 7-11 Atopic dermatitis of the vulva. Atopic dermatitis manifests itself as erythema and scaling in patients who have a history of eczema, nasal allergies, or asthma. Frequently, the presence of accompanying eczema elsewhere on the body aids in the diagnosis. In addition to pruritus, patients may complain of burning, soreness, and even dyspareunia if fissures are present. Careful evaluation is necessary to distinguish this dermatitis from candidal vulvo-vaginitis. (*Courtesy of* L. Edwards, MD.)

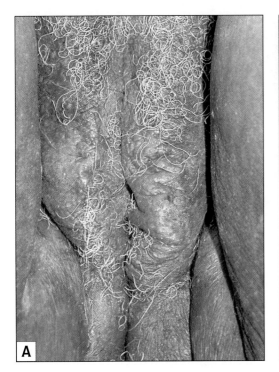

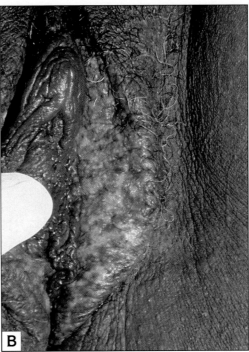

FIGURE 7-12 Lichen simplex chronicus. **A,** This chronic eczematous condition results from habitual rubbing or scratching. It is also termed *neurodermatitis.* It is manifested by hyperpigmentation and lichenification (increased skin markings), which give the affected skin a leathery appearance. **B,** Excoriations and postinflammatory hypopigmentation are other clinical features of lichen simplex chronicus. Trigger factors include an acute flare of atopic dermatitis (as in this patient) or environmental factors, such as irritation from excessive sweating or tight clothing. Candidal infections often can initiate this dermatitis. These initial precipitating conditions may be treated and abate, but pruritus persists and results in an "itch-scratch-itch" cycle. Treatment is challenging and necessitates stopping the scratch-itch cycle. (*Courtesy of* L. Edwards, MD.)

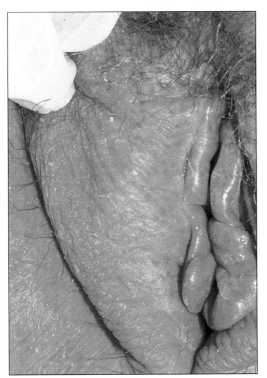

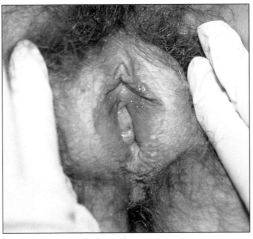

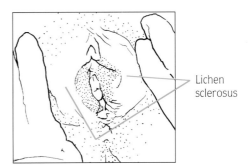

Lichen sclerosus

FIGURE 7-14 Lichen sclerosus of the vulva. This condition presents as hypopigmented papules or as a contiguous plaque (as seen here). Atrophy may cause a crinkled appearance as well as abrasions and purpura. Resorption of the labia minora and contraction of the clitoral hood and introitus may occur in late-stage disease. Intractable pruritus is a common symptom in this condition, even with minimal findings on examination. Lichen sclerosus most often occurs in postmenopausal women and less commonly in prepubertal girls (sometimes misdiagnosed as evidence of sexual abuse). Many of the milder and earlier forms may not be recognized by practitioners and are misdiagnosed as lichen simplex or chronic candida vulvitis.

FIGURE 7-13 Lichen simplex chronicus secondary to a candidal infection. Although the *Candida* infection had been treated successfully and cleared, the initial dermatitis led to a "itch-scratch-itch" cycle, which persisted. The pruritus, usually more intense at night, leads to scratching and results in lichenification, fissures, and even distinct papules and nodules called *prurigo nodularis.* Because of similar symptoms of chronic itching and burning, these patients are sometimes misdiagnosed as having recurrent chronic candidiasis. (*Courtesy of* L. Edwards, MD.)

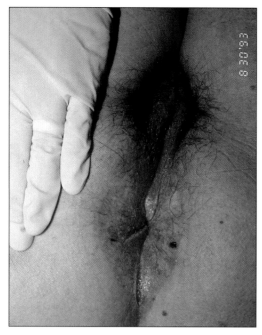

FIGURE 7-15 Distribution of lichen sclerosus. The classic distribution of lichen sclerosus is an hourglass pattern extending from the clitoris down the labia of the vulva and encircling the perianal area. The vaginal mucosa is uninvolved, in contrast to lichen planus, which often involves the vagina.

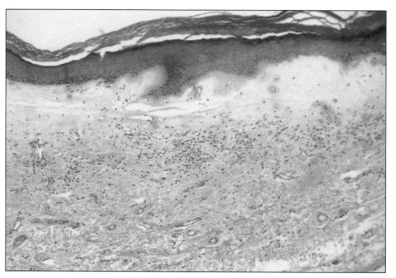

FIGURE 7-16 Histopathologic findings in lichen sclerosus of the vulva. On low-power magnification, there is epidermal atrophy with loss of the normal rete ridge pattern, marked dermal edema, and a bandlike middermal infiltrate. Centrally, there is early bullae formation. Because lichen sclerosus has a distinctive histopathologic appearance, biopsy is extremely helpful in its diagnosis. Once the diagnosis is established, appropriate treatment includes topical corticosteroids and, in some cases, topical testosterone. Increased surveillance of the vulva is necessary because squamous cell carcinoma tends to occur in these individuals. (*Courtesy of* B. Atkinson, MD, and G. Balsara, MD.)

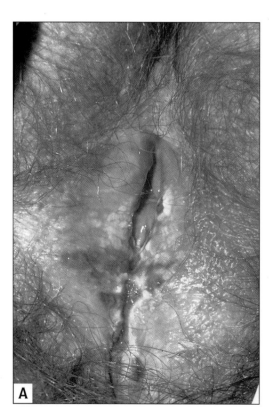

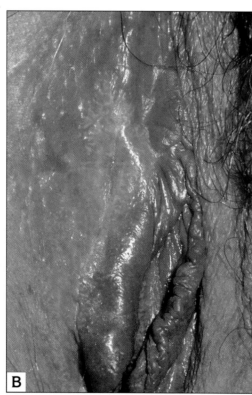

FIGURE 7-17 Lichen planus of the vulva. **A,** Lichen planus is an idiopathic condition that presents as white plaques and erosions. These findings initially may be confused with a candidal infection. **B,** Lichen planus of the vulva. Like the Wickham's striae seen on the oral mucosa, these white, lacy, reticulated plaques on the vulva are specific for lichen planus. On nonmucosal surfaces, lichen planus appears as violaceous, flat-topped, polygonal plaques. Many patients have simultaneous oral and cutaneous disease, but absence of cutaneous plaques does not exclude this diagnosis. (*Courtesy of* L. Edwards, MD.)

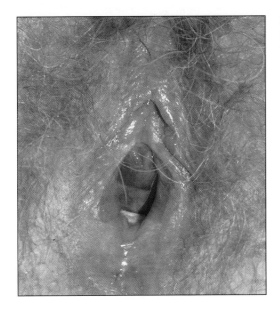

FIGURE 7-18 Lichen planus of the vagina with extensive scarring. Unlike lichen sclerosus, which does not extend into the vagina, lichen planus may cause painful desquamation and, later in disease, fibrosis of the vagina. (*Courtesy of* L. Edwards, MD.)

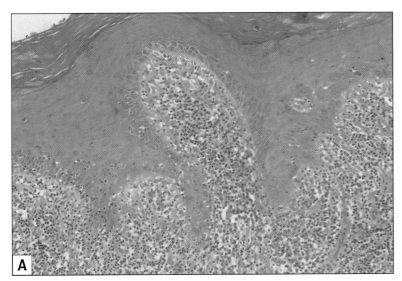

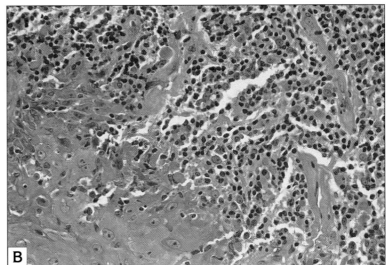

FIGURE 7-19 Histopathologic findings in lichen planus of the vulva. Clinical diagnosis of lichen planus is frequently delayed. Patients may complain of intense dysparenunia and purulent discharge, which is often misdiagnosed as trichomoniasis or atrophic or candidal vaginitis. Biopsy can be helpful in establishing the correct diagnosis. **A,** On midpower magnification, there is hyperkeratosis and epidermal hyperplasia with a sawtooth configuration of the rete ridges (downward projections of the lower epidermis). There is a dense bandlike inflammatory infiltrate along the interface between the epidermis and dermis. **B,** On high-power magnification, Civatte or colloid bodies appear in the lower epidermis and upper dermis as homogeneously, eosinophilic round structures. They represent degenerated keratinocytes and are commonly seen in lichen planus. (*Courtesy of* B. Atkinson, MD, and G. Balsara, MD.)

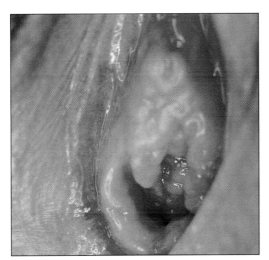

FIGURE 7-20 Vulvar vestibulitis. Vulvar vestibulitis is a chronic clinical syndrome manifested by significant pain on vaginal entry or vestibular touch, localized tenderness to pressure within the vestibule, and variable degrees of vestibular erythema [3]. Confluent erythema involving the entire vestibule is shown here in a patient with vestibulitis. In other patients, erythema may be absent or localized to the Bartholin's glands and the paraurethral Skene's glands. (*Courtesy of* M. Spence, MD.)

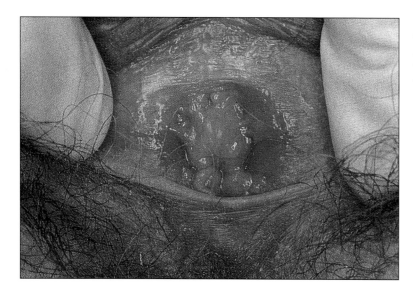

FIGURE 7-21 Vulvar vestibulitis presenting with erythema around the Bartholin's glands. The openings of these glands are seen at 5 and 7 o'clock. Patients may complain of dyspareunia, pain with tampon insertion, or dysuria. In establishing the diagnosis, urinary tract and vulvovaginal infection should first be ruled out. (*From* Leibowitch *et al.* [4]; with permission.)

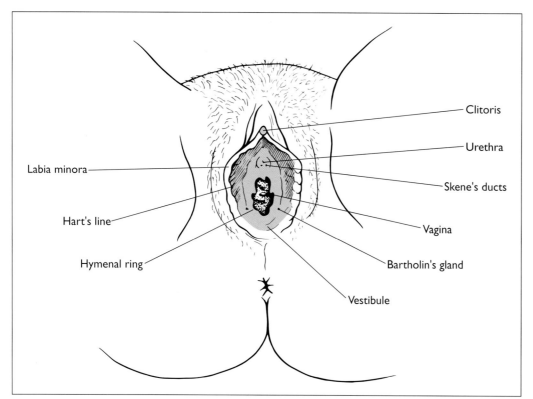

FIGURE 7-22 Schematic drawing of the vulvar vestibule. The vulvar vestibule is the portion of the vulva extending from the inner portion of the labia minora, beginning at Hart's line, to the hymen.

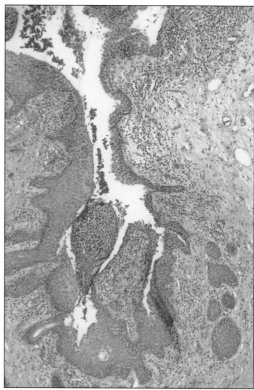

FIGURE 7-23 Histopathologic findings in vulvar vestibulitis. There is squamous metaplasia of the vestibular gland epithelium and a chronic inflammatory infiltrate. The criteria for diagnosis of vulvar vestibulitis are clinical; the pathology is often nonspecific. (*Courtesy of* B. Atkinson, MD, and G. Balsara, MD.)

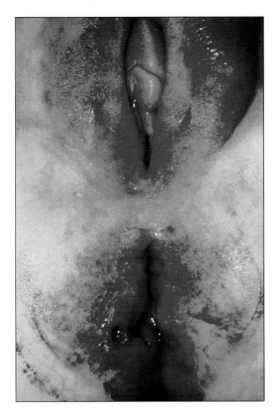

FIGURE 7-24 Crohn's disease of the vulva and perianal area. Crohn's disease most commonly involves the perianal and perineal skin by direct extension of suppurating granulomas forming abscesses or draining fistulas. More rarely, noncontiguous or "metastatic" involvement may occur, manifesting as nodules and linear fissures in intertriginous folds ("knife-cut" sign). In this patient, there is extension of the disease to the labia majora. Most patients with anogenital lesions already carry a diagnosis of Crohn's disease or at least have symptoms of diarrhea and abdominal pain. The differential diagnosis includes granuloma inguinale as well as granulomatous disease seen with fungal and mycobacterial infections. (*Courtesy of* B. Cohen, MD; *from* American Academy of Dermatology [1], with permission.)

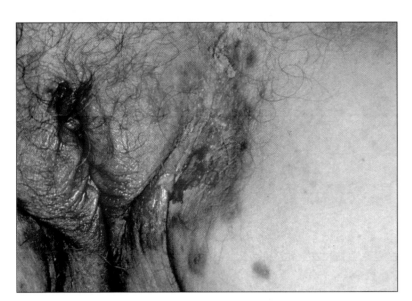

FIGURE 7-25 Toxic epidermal necrolysis (TEN) of the groin. TEN is believed to represent a hypersensitivity reaction to a medication or infection. It results in widespread sloughing of cutaneous and mucosal surfaces. However, it may present initially as a nonspecific erythema of the labia that progresses to an erosive vulvitis. The lesions in this patient were initially thought to be satellite lesions of candidiasis, but biopsy showed subepidermal bullae formation characteristic of TEN. (*Courtesy of* M. Turner, MD; *from* American Academy of Dermatology [1]; with permission.)

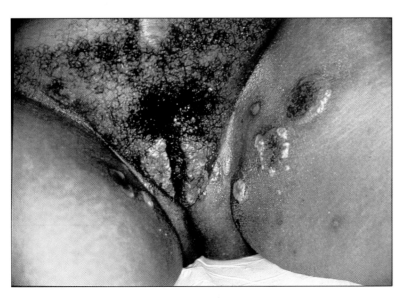

FIGURE 7-26 Pemphigus vulgaris. This autoimmune bullous disease typically involves cutaneous surfaces but may be preceded or accompanied by mucosal involvement. Patients may present first with painful oral and genital lesions, and infectious etiologies need to be considered and excluded. Diagnosis can be established by biopsy with histologic and immunofluorescence testing. Bullous lesions of pemphigus in the vulva may erode or assume a vegetative appearance. Because there is a breach in the normal integrity of skin and mucosa, there is a high risk for superinfection. In advanced disease, scarring and adhesions may occur in the vulvar area but do not occur on cutaneous surfaces. (*Courtesy of* M. Turner, MD; *from* American Academy of Dermatology [1], with permission.)

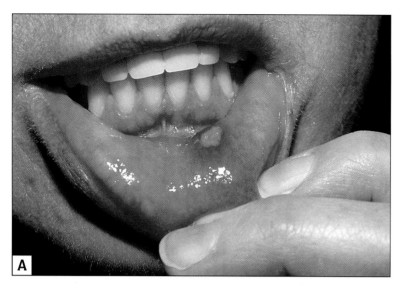

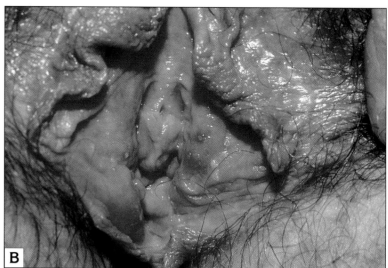

FIGURE 7-27 Oral and genital ulcers of Behçet's disease. **A** and **B**, Behçet's disease is characterized by the triad of recurrent oral ulcers, recurrent genital ulcers, and uveitis. The oral and vulvar aphthae present as tender, shallow, punched-out ulcers. Anogenital involvement is seen in about 90% of affected patients. The differential diagnosis of these vulvar lesions includes herpes and chancroid. Vulvar aphthae may also be found in association with inflammatory bowel disease or as an idiopathic phenomenon in the absence of systemic disease.

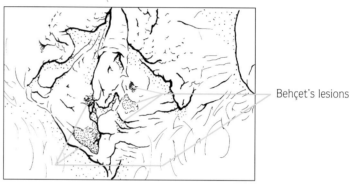

Behçet's lesions

FIGURE 7-28 Differential diagnosis of vulvar ulcers.

Differential diagnosis of vulvar ulcers

Infectious	Noninfectious
Primary syphilis	Aphthous ulcers
Chancroid	Idiopathic HIV
Granuloma inguinale	Behçet's disease
Lymphogranuloma venereum	Crohn's disease
Herpes simplex	Neoplasms (basal cell carcinoma, squamous cell carcinoma)

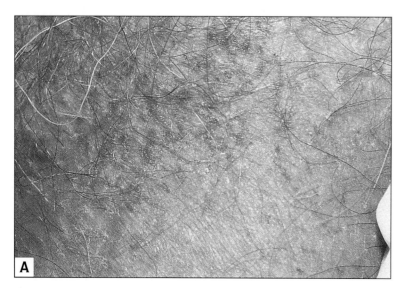

FIGURE 7-29 Steroid atrophy. Although corticosteroids are useful for a variety of vulvar dermatoses, their use can result in atrophy. **A**, The skin may appear shiny and thin with telangiectasis. (*continued*)

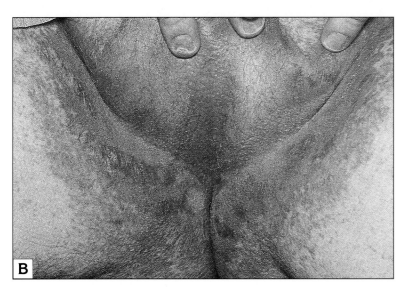

FIGURE 7-29 (*continued*) **B.** Striae may develop. Low-potency topical corticosteroids should generally be used in the genital area, although medium and high-potency steroids may be necessary for conditions such as chronic eczematous dermatitis and lichen sclerosus. The vulvar area should be monitored carefully for signs of atrophy, particularly with a prolonged course of treatment. (*From* Lynch and Edwards [2]; with permission.)

INFECTIOUS VULVITIS

Candidal Infections

Differential diagnostic features of vaginitis in adult women

Feature	Normal	Candida vaginitis	Bacterial vaginosis	Trichomonal vaginitis
Symptoms	None or physiologic leukorrhea	Vulvar pruritus, soreness, ↑ discharge, dysuria, dyspareunia	Moderate malodorous discharge	Profuse, purulent, offensive discharge; pruritus; dyspareunia
Discharge				
Amount	Scant to moderate	Scant to moderate	Moderate	Profuse
Color	Clear or white	White	White or gray	Yellow
Consistency	Floccular, nonhomogeneous	Clumped but variable	Homogeneous, uniformly coating walls	Homogenous
Bubbles	Absent	Absent	Present	Present
Appearance of vulva and vagina	Normal	Introital and vulvar erythema, edema, occasional pustules, vaginal erythema	No inflammation	Erythema and swelling of vulvar and vaginal epithelium, "strawberry" cervix
pH of vaginal fluid	< 4.5	< 4.5	> 4.7	5–6.0
Amine test (16% KOH)	Negative	Negative	Positive	Occasionally present
Saline microscopy	Normal epithelial cells, lactobacilli predominate	Normal flora, blastospores (yeast) 40%–50%, pseudohyphae	Clue cells, coccobacillary flora predominate, absence of leukocytes, motile curved rods	PMNs +++, motile trichomonads (80%–90%), no clue cells or abnormal flora
10% KOH microscopy	Negative	Positive (60%–90%)	Negative (except in mixed infections)	Negative

KOH—potassium hydroxide; PMNs—polymorphonuclear cells.

FIGURE 7-30 Clinical and laboratory features of candidal, bacterial, and trichomonal vaginitis in adult women. Women who complain of abnormal discharge or vulvar discomfort should be evaluated for vaginitis. Vaginal discharge associated with vaginitis can act as an irritant to the vulva causing erythema and pain. (*Adapted from* Sobel [5].)

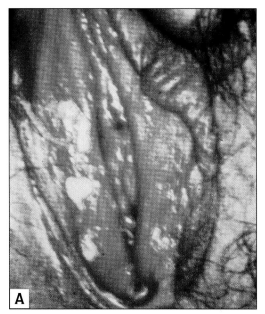

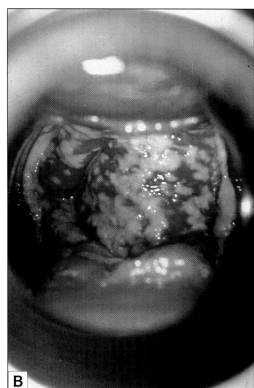

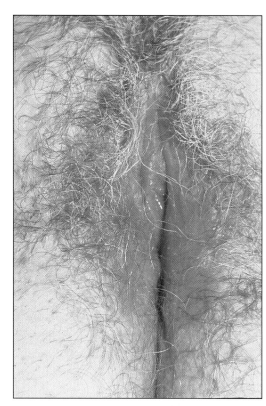

FIGURE 7-31 Vulvovaginal candidiasis.
A, Erythema and discrete areas of white, cheesy discharge are seen on the vulva. There is often associated pruritus, soreness, and dyspareunia. A subset of patients have chronic recurrent candidiasis, which may require a course of oral antifungal therapy. **B**, "Characteristic" cheesy discharge of vulvovaginal candidiasis, seen here on speculum examination, is found in a minority of patients. (Panel 31A *courtesy of* E. Hernandez, MD; panel 31B *courtesy of* J.D. Sobel, MD).

FIGURE 7-32 Candidal infection causing "beefy" red appearance of the vulva. (*Courtesy of* L. Edwards, MD.)

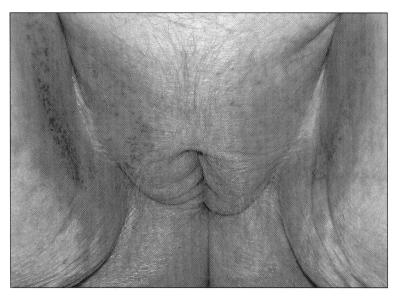

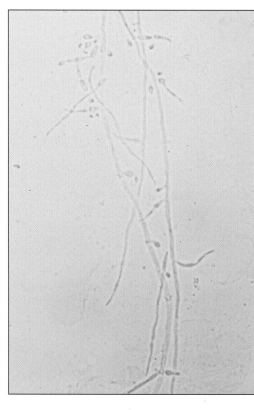

FIGURE 7-34 Pseudohyphae and spores of *Candida* on Gram stain. Potassium hydroxide 10% is the preferred diagnostic method.

FIGURE 7-33 Vulvovaginal candidiasis involving the entire perineal area and labiocrural fold in a patient with diabetes. The erosions present bilaterally are due to scratching. Satellite lesions, as seen here on the inner thighs and mons pubis, are typical. Predisposing factors to candidal infections include high estrogen states (such as pregnancy), diabetes mellitus, corticosteroid therapy, antibiotics, and HIV infection. (*Courtesy of* L. Edwards, MD.)

Differential diagnosis of candidal vulvovaginitis/vulvitis

Infectious: bacterial, trichomonal (discharge can cause a
 reddened, inflamed vulva)
Eczema, psoriasis (these dermatoses affect vulvar but *not*
 vaginal tissue; can be confused with candidal vulvitis)
Intertrigo (irritation in labial folds due to friction and moisture)
Vulvar vestibulitis-idiopathic
Hypersensitivity or allergic vulvovaginitis
Chemical, irritant vulvovaginitis
Physiologic desquamation of epithelium creating white
 discharge in/from vagina or whitened areas in labial folds
 (smegma)

FIGURE 7-35 Differential diagnosis of candidal vulvovaginitis/
vulvitis.

Treatment of candidal vulvovaginitis

Topical (creams, suppositories)
 Nystatin (azoles are preferable)
 Azoles: clotrimazole (Gyne-lotrimin), miconazole (Monistat),
  butoconazole (Femstat), terconazole (Terazol), tioconazole
  (Vagistat)
Oral
 Ketoconazole (Nizoral)
 Fluconazole (Diflucan)
 Itraconazole (Sporonox)

FIGURE 7-36 Treatment of candidal vulvovaginitis. Fluconazole,
150 mg orally, may be effective as a single dose treatment for
candidal vaginitis. Patients with recurrent infections may benefit
from prophylaxis with repeated use of a topical or oral agent.

Bacterial Infections

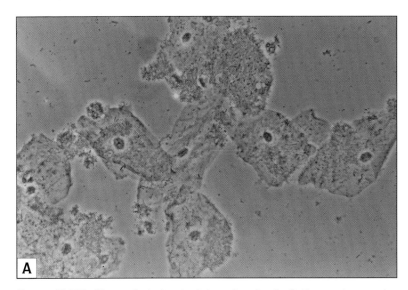

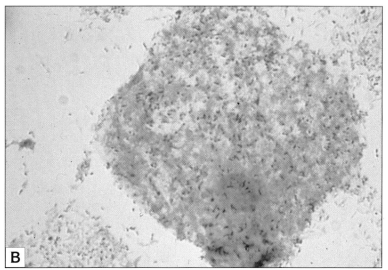

FIGURE 7-37 Clue cells in bacterial vaginosis. **A,** Saline wet mount
showing typical "clue cells," typified by the stippled appearance of
the epithelial cells due to the presence of coccobacilli (*arrows*).
Lactobacilli and white blood cells, which are normally present, are
absent. **B,** Gram stain of a typical clue cell as seen in bacterial vaginosis demonstrates gram-negative bacilli studding the epithelial
cell. Most patients who present with bacterial vaginosis complain of
a discharge that has a fishy odor. Some experience itching or pain
from the discharge causing an irritant dermatitis. (Panel 37A *courtesy of* S.L. Hillier, PhD; panel 37B *courtesy of* J.D. Sobel, MD.)

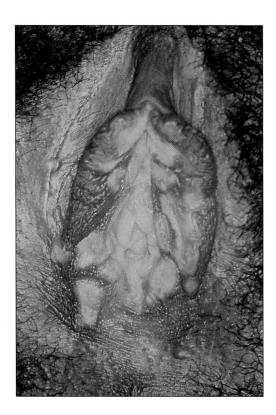

FIGURE 7-38
Condyloma lata. These "moist papules" of secondary syphilis are highly infectious. They appear as multiple white or gray hypertrophic papules and nodules. The primary syphilitic chancre is a painless ulcer with a raised border and clean base, usually accompanied by regional lymphadenopathy. Occasionally, the primary and secondary lesions overlap in time.

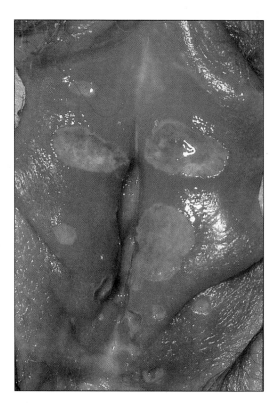

FIGURE 7-39
Chancroid. These single or multiple painful ulcers, with ragged edges and necrotic bases, are caused by *Haemophilus ducreyi*, a gram-negative bacillus. (*Courtesy of* A. Hood, MD; *from* American Academy of Dermatology [1]; with permission.)

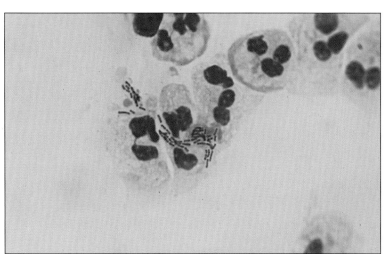

FIGURE 7-40 *Haemophilus ducreyi*, causative organism of chancroid. *H. ducreyi* can be detected by the deep staining of the two ends of the organism ("closed safety pin") as well as by its appearance extracellularly in rows ("school of fish"), as seen here. (*Courtesy of* E.J. Bottone, PhD.)

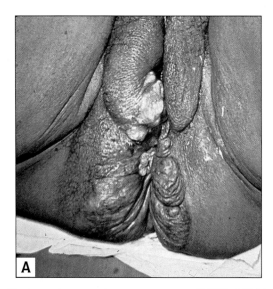

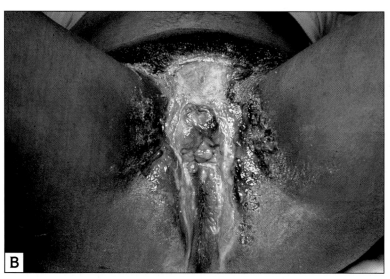

FIGURE 7-41 Lymphogranuloma venereum (LGV). LGV is a sexually transmitted disease caused by *Chlamydia trachomatis*. Infection travels from the site of inoculation to involve the regional lymph nodes. The depression caused by Pupart's ligament with enlarged inguinal lymph nodes above and below is called the *groove sign*. **A**, The edematous and fibrotic external genitalia of a patient with chronic LGV. **B**, Vulva of the same patient with chronic LGV 6 weeks postoperatively after scarred and damaged tissue has been excised. (*Courtesy of* M. Spence, MD.)

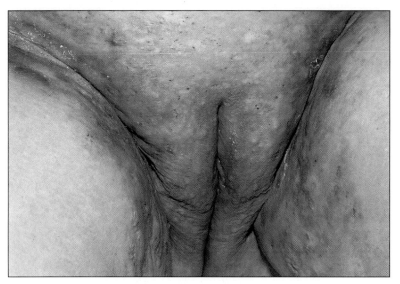

FIGURE 7-42 Hidradenitis suppurativa. This is a chronic inflammatory disease of the apocrine glands, which are numerous in the vulva and axillae. The primary event in the pathogenesis of this disorder is not infection but rather occlusion of apocrine glands and their associated hair follicles. However, this is often followed by secondary bacterial superinfection. The process eventually may result in widespread and disfiguring fibrosis. It is most common in women aged 20 to 40 years. Shown here are multiple abscesslike nodules and scarring of the vulvar area.

Parasitic Infections

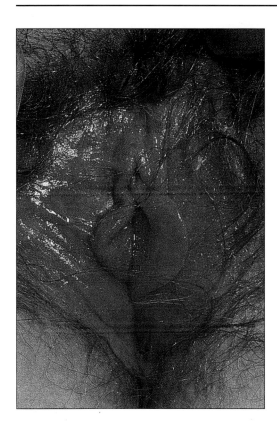

FIGURE 7-43 *Trichomonas vaginalis* vaginitis. Erythema and inflammation of the vulva caused by the inflammatory discharge in a patient with trichomonas vaginitis. (*From* Leibowitch *et al.* [4], with permission.)

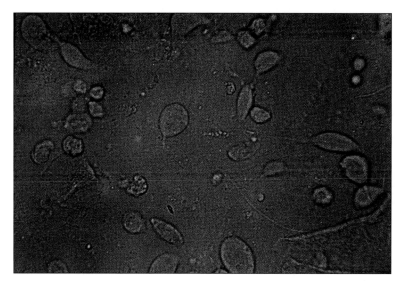

FIGURE 7-44 Saline wet mount demonstrating motile, oval, or pear-shaped trichomonads seen with *Trichomonas vaginalis* vaginitis. (*From* Tovell and Young [6]; with permission.)

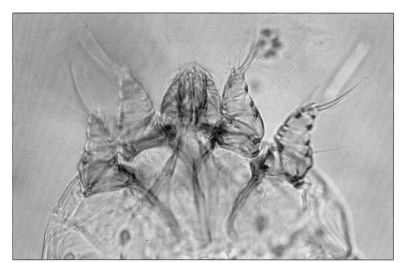

FIGURE 7-45 *Sarcoptes scabiei*, causative organism of scabies. Scabies causes an intensely pruritic eruption, with lesions especially prominent in the webspaces of finger and toes and in the genital and buttock area. The female mite burrows into the stratum corneum of the skin and deposits her eggs, causing a hypersensitivity reaction. (*Courtesy of* L. Duncan, MD.)

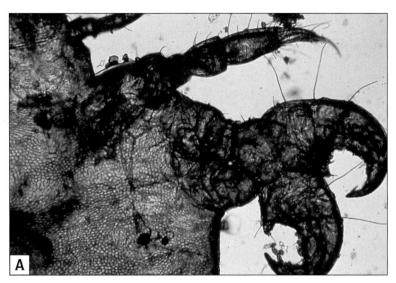

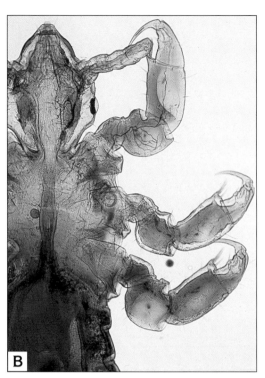

FIGURE 7-46 Human lice. **A**, *Phthirus pubis* is the causative organism of pediculosis pubis. This crablike louse, which is sexually transmitted, lives selectively in the pubic area and deposits its eggs or nits on pubic hair. **B**, The contrasting appearance of the louse that causes pediculosis capitis (head lice). (*Courtesy of* L. Duncan, MD.)

Viral Infections

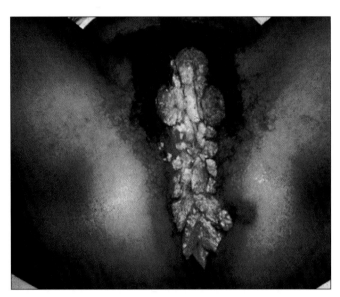

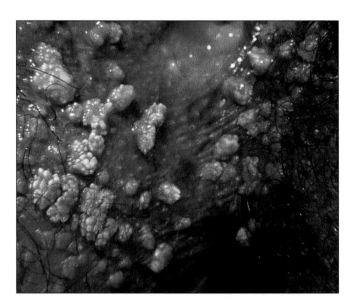

FIGURE 7-47 Condyloma acuminata. Multiple white hyperkeratotic pedunculated verrucae clustered on the keratinized portion of the vulva. Condylomata on the nonkeratinized mucosal surfaces of the vulva have a flesh-colored moist appearance. These genital warts are caused by the human papillomavirus (HPV), which is usually transmitted by sexual contact. HPV type 6 and 11 are common subtypes causing infection in the vulvar area. Certain subtypes, such as HPV type 16 and 18, which cause genital flat warts, have been associated with cervical dysplasia and carcinoma. Modalities to treat condyloma include cryotherapy, podophyllin, trichloroacetic acid and laser therapy. (*Courtesy of* M. Spence, MD.)

FIGURE 7-48 Close-up view of condyloma acuminata with multiple, pedunculated, and sessile venereal warts. (*From* Tovell and Young [6]; with permission.)

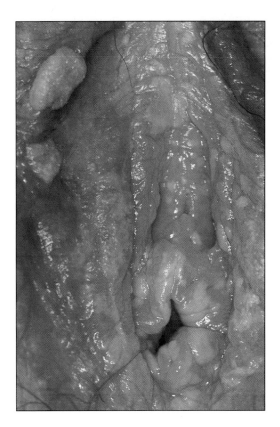

FIGURE 7-49 Multiple human papillomavirus lesions demonstrated with acetowhitening. When warts are indistinct, diagnosis is aided by acetowhitening with vinegar or 5% acetic acid. Vinegar applied to the area for approximately 5 minutes causes dehydration of the keratin of the condyloma, and they appear whitened and more easily identified. (*Courtesy of* R. Reid, MD.)

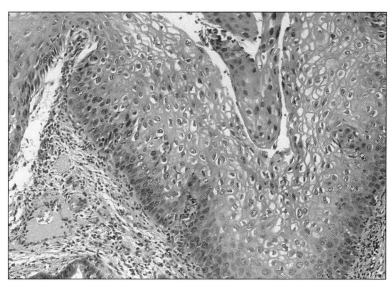

FIGURE 7-50 Histopathologic findings in condyloma acuminata. There is prominent koilocytosis of the epidermal cells with perinuclear vacuolization and crinkled, hyperchromatic nuclei. These changes are more marked in the valley of the epidermis than the peaks. (*Courtesy of* B. Atkinson, MD, and G. Balsara, MD.)

FIGURE 7-51 Human papillomavirus types associated with vulvar presentations.

HPV types associated with vulvar presentations

Disease	Clinical manifestation	HPV type
Condylomata acuminata	Exophytic lesions	6,11
Cervical, vaginal, vulvar flat warts	Shiny patches, irregular surface	16,18
Cervical intraepithelial neoplasia	May not be visualized with naked eye; detected by colposcopy, Papanicolaou smear	16,18,31,33,35

HPV—human papillomavirus.

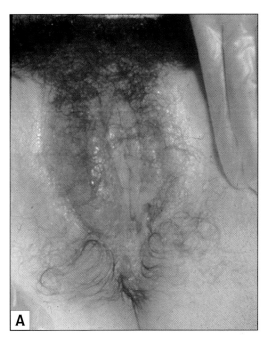

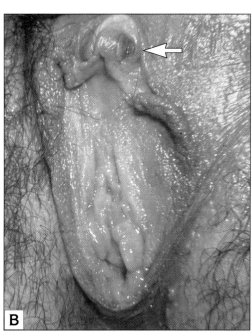

FIGURE 7-52 Herpes vulvitis. **A**, Primary herpes simplex virus (HSV) infection begins with vesicles that rupture and develop into painful erosions. Erythema and edema, as shown here on the vulva, are also seen. The vagina and cervix can be involved, and patients may feel systemically ill. **B**, Recurrent HSV infections tend to be less severe and may sometimes be asymptomatic. Recurrent episodes may be preceded by a prodrome of tingling or burning in the area. A localized erosive HSV infection involving the clitoris is shown here (*arrow*). (*Courtesy of* M. Spence, MD.)

A

B

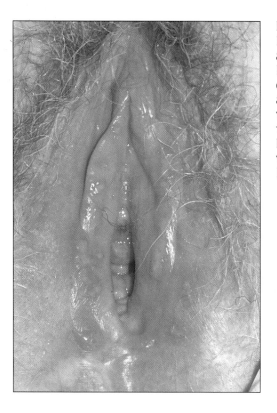

FIGURE 7-53
Herpes simplex affecting the vulva. Erosions on an erythematous base arising from broken vesicles are clustered in several locations on the vulva. (*Courtesy of* L. Edwards, MD.)

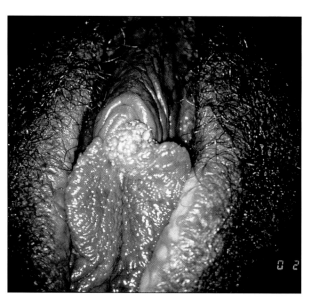

FIGURE 7-54 Coinfection of herpes simplex and condyloma acuminata affecting the vulva. Herpes simplex virus erosions surrounded by erythema are seen on the left labia. Another sexually transmitted disease, human papillomavirus–induced condylomata involve the superior aspect of the labia. (*Courtesy of* E. Hernandez, MD.)

FIGURE 7-55 Tzanck preparation using Giemsa stain showing multinucleated giant cells in herpesvirus infection. The giant cells represent keratinocytes infected with the herpes virus.

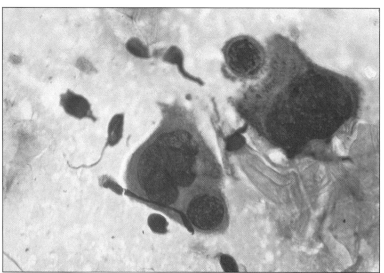

FIGURE 7-56 A and **B**, HIV ulcers affecting the vulva. (*Courtesy of* J.D. Sobel, MD)

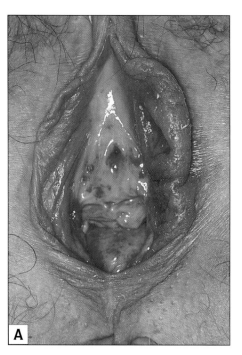

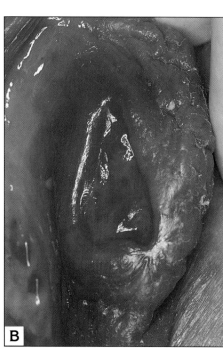

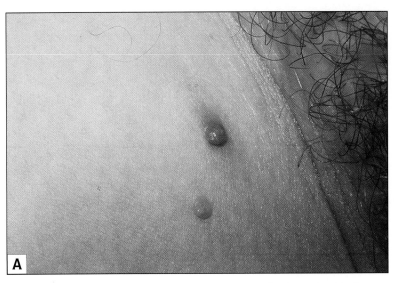

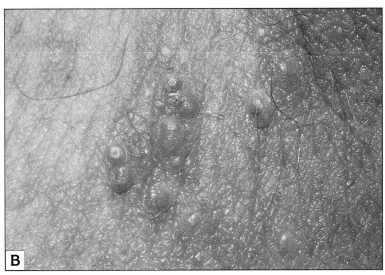

FIGURE 7-57 Molluscum contagiosum. **A** and **B**, This viral infection presents as multiple, pink or flesh-colored, dome-shaped papules with central umbilication. It is caused by a pox virus that is sexually transmitted in adults. (*Courtesy of* L. Edwards, MD.)

NEOPLASMS OF THE VULVA

Malignant Lesions

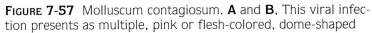

Vulvar neoplasms

Vulvar intraepithelial neoplasia
  Squamous
  Nonsquamous
Invasive squamous cell carcinoma
Verrucous carcinoma of Buschke-Löwenstein
Basal cell carcinoma
Melanoma

FIGURE 7-58 Vulvar neoplasms.

Classification of VIN

Squamous
  VIN 1 (mild dysplasia)
  VIN 2 (moderate dysplasia)
  VIN 3 (severe dysplasia or carcinoma in situ)
Nonsquamous
  Paget's disease
  Melanoma in situ

VIN—vulvar intraepithelial neoplasia.

FIGURE 7-59 Classification of vulvar intraepithelial neoplasia [7].

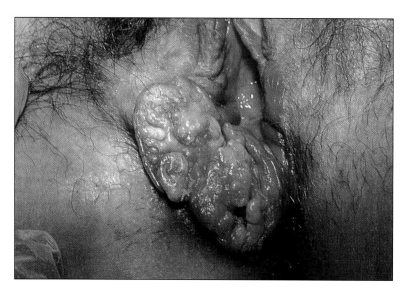

FIGURE 7-60 Cauliflower-like verrucous squamous cell carcinoma of Bushke-Löwenstein. These lesions appear as large nodules that may have a smooth or cauliflower-like surface. These "giant warts" have been linked to human papillomavirus. (*From* Leibowitch *et al.* [4]; with permission.)

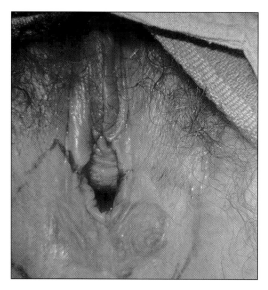

FIGURE 7-61 Vulvar intraepithelial neoplasia (VIN) 3 in the perineum. VIN 3, or squamous cell carcinoma in situ, appears here as a pink plaque with accentuated skin markings and well-defined borders. The color of the lesion may also be white, particularly on the keratinized epithelium of the vulva. (*Courtesy of* E. Hernandez, MD.)

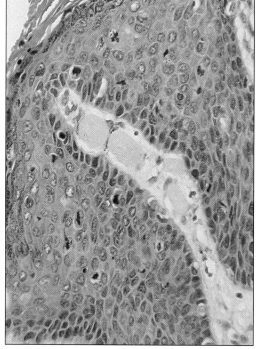

FIGURE 7-62 Histopathologic examination of vulvar intraepithelial neoplasia 3 (squamous cell carcinoma in situ). High-power magnification shows acanthosis (epidermal thickening), loss of polarity of maturation in the epidermis, and dyskeratosis (eosinophilic epidermal cells due to abnormal keratinization). Full-thickness atypia of keratinocytes is present. (*Courtesy of* B. Atkinson, MD, and G. Balsara, MD.)

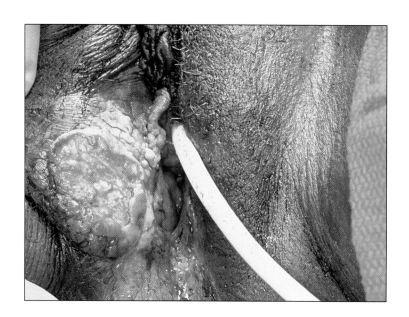

FIGURE 7-63 Squamous cell carcinoma of the vulva manifested by a large, exophytic polypoid nodule on the right labia majora. Squamous cell carcinoma is the most common vulvar malignancy. It generally occurs in women above age 60 years. (*Courtesy of* E. Hernandez, MD.)

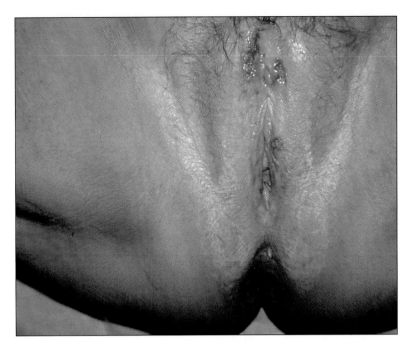

FIGURE 7-64 Squamous cell carcinoma, appearing as an ulcerated plaque on the prepuce, arising in a background of lichen sclerosus. The increased risk of squamous cell carcinoma in patients with lichen sclerosus necessitates their close supervision and biopsy of suspicious lesions. (*Courtesy of* E. Hernandez, MD.)

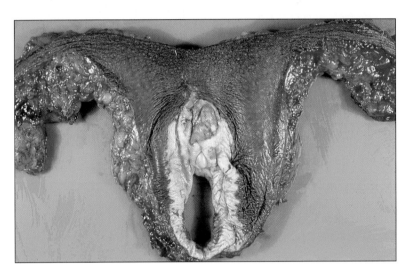

FIGURE 7-65 Pathologic specimen of excised vulva demonstrating squamous cell carcinoma and vitiligo. The specimen demonstrates two coincident pathologic processes. The squamous cell carcinoma located above the prepuce necessitated the vulvectomy. The specimen also reveals an unrelated condition, vitiligo. Vitiligo is an idiopathic process in which melanocytes are lost from the skin, probably due to an autoimmune process. Clinically, these appear as white macules with a predisposition to periorificial areas such as the vulva. (*Courtesy of* E. Hernandez, MD.)

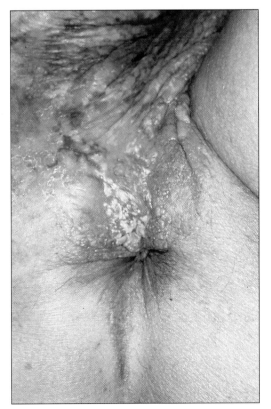

FIGURE 7-66 Vulvar Paget's disease is usually an extension from anal and perianal disease. It presents as a pruritic erythematous, irregular plaque with occasionally white patches that can often be mistaken for an excoriated eczematous lesion; there is a correlation with adnexal carcinomas and internal malignancies. (*Courtesy of* M. Turner, MD; *from* American Academy of Dermatology [1], with permission.)

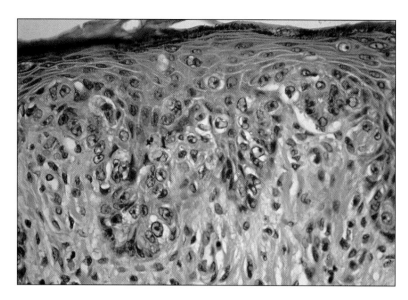

FIGURE 7-67 Histopathologic findings in extramammary Paget's disease of the vulva. High-power magnification shows that Paget's cells are present throughout the full thickness of the epidermis. They are pale cells with large nuclei, which resemble epithelial cells but lack intercellular bridges. (*Courtesy of* B. Atkinson, MD, and G. Balsara, MD.)

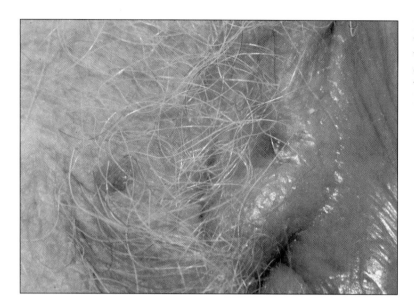

FIGURE 7-68 Two pigmented basal cell carcinomas of the vulva following radiation therapy to the area. These carcinomas, which arise from the basal cells of the epidermis, typically occur on sun-exposed skin. They rarely occur on the vulva, except in the setting of radiation, thermal burns, and scars. (*Courtesy of* L. Edwards, MD.)

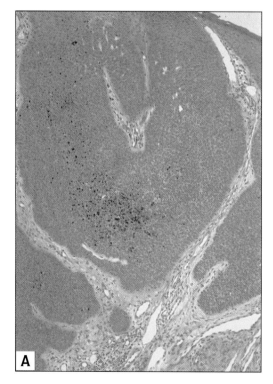

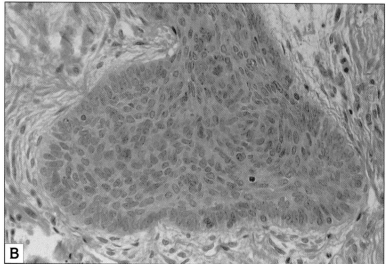

FIGURE 7-69 Histopathologic findings in basal cell carcinoma of vulva. **A**, On low-power magnification, there are masses of different sizes, representing proliferating basaloid cells. **B**, On high-power magnification, there is peripheral palisading of the basal cell layer and focal cell necrosis. (*Courtesy of* B. Atkinson, MD, and G. Balsara, MD.)

Pigmented Lesions of the Vulva

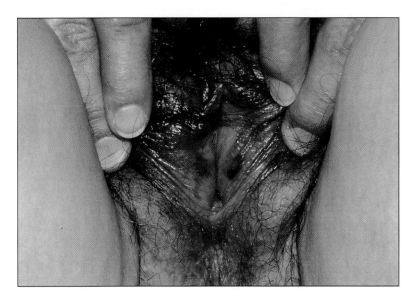

FIGURE 7-70 Vulvar melanosis appearing as darkly pigmented, irregular macules on the labia minora. These benign lesions are clinically distinguished from lentigines by their larger size and irregular borders. These features can mimic melanoma, and biopsy may be necessary. Histologically, vulvar melanosis demonstrates intense basal cell hyperpigmentation but lacks melanocyte atypia.

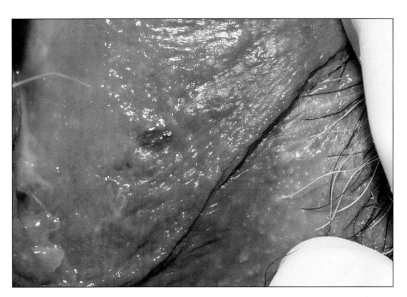

FIGURE 7-71 Junctional nevus of the vulva appearing as a small, homogeneously gray macule with sharply defined borders. An estimated 2% of women have nevi located on the vulva. The nevus pictured here is benign. However, dysplastic nevi and melanoma can occur on the vulva. Therefore, pigmented lesions that are changing or have clinically atypical features (*eg*, pigment variegation, irregular borders) warrant close evaluation and, frequently, excision. (*Courtesy of* L. Edwards, MD.)

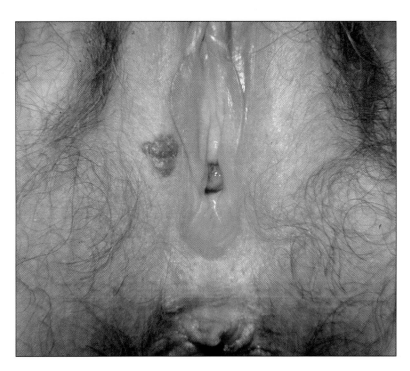

FIGURE 7-72 Malignant melanoma of the vulva. The lesion is a gray-black plaque with irregular borders on the right labia majora. Approximately 2% to 5% of melanomas occur on the vulva. Vulvar melanomas have a poorer prognosis than melanoma of the torso, reflecting their tendency to be thicker and more advanced at the time of diagnosis. (*Courtesy of* E. Hernandez, MD.)

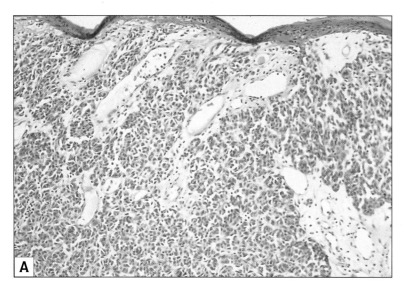

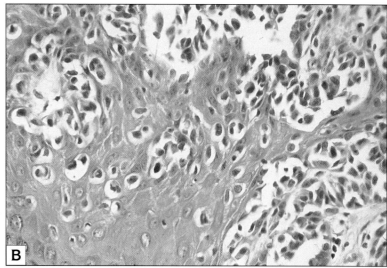

FIGURE 7-73 Histopathologic findings in malignant melanoma of the vulva. **A**, Low-power magnification shows melanoma in the vertical growth phase, with a proliferation of small melanoma cells extending from the epidermis into the dermis in nests and sheets. There is also associated vascular ectasia. **B**, On higher magnification, there are nests of melanoma cells as well as pagetoid (single-cell) melanoma cells that are present throughout the epidermis. There is also individual cell necrosis present. (*Courtesy of* B. Atkinson, MD, and G. Balsara, MD.)

VULVODYNIA

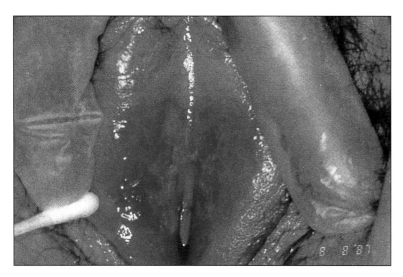

FIGURE 7-74 Vulvodynia. Vulvodynia, or "burning vulva syndrome," is a clinical syndrome defined by chronic pain or burning, often with minimal physical findings. Vulvar vestibulitis is one subset. It can present with erythemas, as pictured here.

Classification and treatment of vulvodynia

Subset	Therapeutic options
Vulvar vestibulitis	Surgical excision
	Alpha-interferon injections
Cyclic vulvitis	Empiric anticandida therapy
Dysesthetic vulvodynia	Low-dose amitriptyline desipramine

FIGURE 7-75 Classification and treatment of vulvodynia. Subsets of vulvodynia are delineated by patterns of pain, exacerbating factors, and response to treatment. These include vulvar vestibulitis (*see* Figs. 7-20 to 7-23), cyclic vulvitis (intermittent pain often with menstruation, possibly related to candida), and dysesthetic vulvodynia (possibly a neuralgia). Initial management entails avoidance of irritating contacts as well as identification and treatment of any coexisting dermatoses or infections. Therapeutic options are often limited and unsatisfactory.

REFERENCES

1. Turner ML: Vulvar diseases. *In* Schosser RH (ed.): American Academy of Dermatology: *National Library of Dermatologic Teaching Slides*. Evanston, IL: American Academy of Dermatology; 1988.

2. Lynch PJ, Edwards L: *Genital Dermatology*. New York: Churchill Livingstone; 1994.

3. McKay M, Frankman O, Horowitz BJ, *et al.*: Vulvar vestibulitis and vestibular papillomatosis: Report of the ISSVD Committee on Vulvodynia. *J Reprod Med* 1991, 36:413.

4. Leibowitch M, Staughton R, Neill S, *et al.*: *An Atlas of Vulval Disease: A Combined Dermatological, Gynaecological and Venereological Approach*. London: Martin Dunitz; 1995.

5. Sobel JD: Vaginal infections in adult women. *Med Clin North Am* 1990, 74:1576.

6. Tovell HMM, Young AW Jr: *Diseases of the Vulva in Clinical Practice*. New York: Elsevier; 1991.

7. Wilkinson EJ, Kneale B, Lynch PJ: Report of the ISSVD Terminology Committee. *J Reprod Med* 1986, 31:973–974.

SELECTED BIBLIOGRAPHY

Kaye ET: Diseases of the vulva. *In* Carr P, Freund K (eds.): *Primary Care of Women*. Philadelphia: W.B. Saunders; 1995.

Leibowitch M, Staughton R, Neill S, *et al.*: *An Atlas of Vulval Disease: A Combined Dermatological, Gynaecological and Venereological Approach*. London: Martin Dunitz; 1995.

Lynch PJ, Edwards L: *Genital Dermatology*. New York: Churchill Livingstone; 1994.

Tovell HMM, Young AW: *Diseases of the Vulva in Clinical Practice*. New York: Elsevier Science Publishing; 1991.

Turner MLC, Marinoff SC (eds.): General principles in the diagnosis and treatment of vulvar diseases. *Dermatol Clin* 1992, 10:275–281.

CHAPTER 8

Cervicitis and Endometritis

David E. Soper

NORMAL CERVICAL ANATOMY

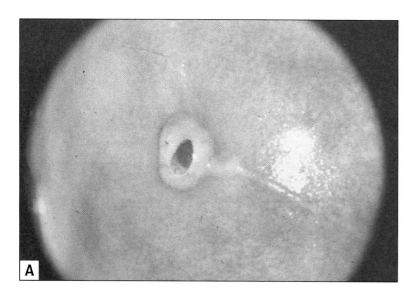

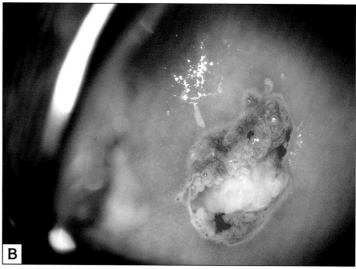

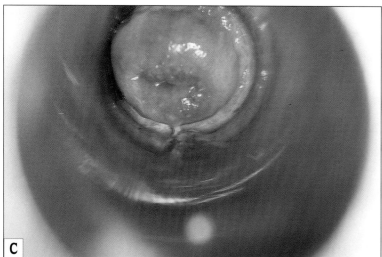

FIGURE 8-1 Clinical views of the normal cervix. **A,** Nulliparous. The external cervical os is round and small in a nulliparous woman. **B,** Multiparous. The external cervical os is wider and the squamocolumnar junction more easily visualized on the multiparous cervix. **C,** Multiparous cervix following vaginal delivery. The external cervical os is wider and more "fish-mouth" in appearance following vaginal delivery. (Panel 1A *from* American College of Obstetrics and Gynecology [1], with permission; panel 1C *courtesy of* O. Williamson, MD.)

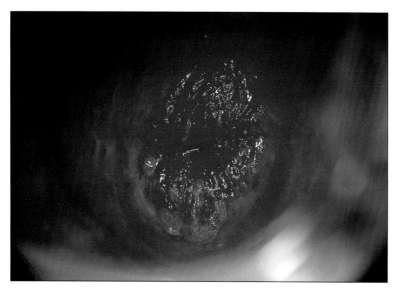

FIGURE 8-2 Cervical ectopy. The eversion of the endocervical columnar cells causes the normal finding of "ectopy." This commonly occurs in women on oral contraceptives. Cervical ectopy may predispose women to infection with *Chlamydia* [2]. (*Courtesy of* P. Wolner-Hanssen, MD.)

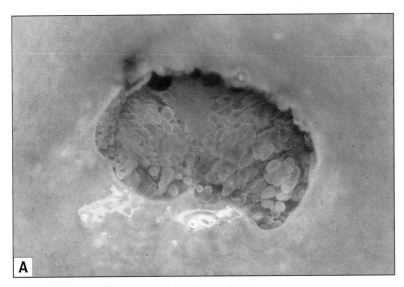

FIGURE 8-3 Squamocolumnar junction. **A** and **B,** Colpophoto-graphs showing a normal squamocolumnar junction. The flat-appearing squamous cells of the ectocervix meet the taller, glan-dular-appearing columnar epithelial cells of the endocervix at this junction. **C,** Diagram of the normal squamocolumnar junction. The squamocolumnar junction is the vulnerable site of the cervix with respect to the origin of human papillomavirus–induced dysplastic change. (Panel 3A *courtesy of* D. Townsend, MD.)

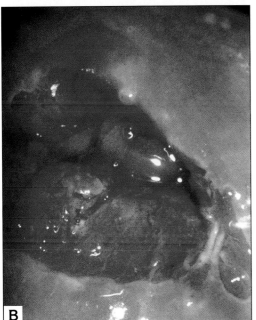

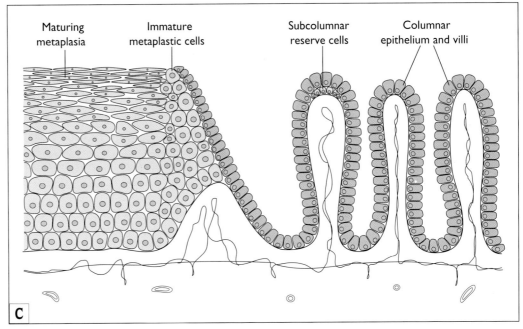

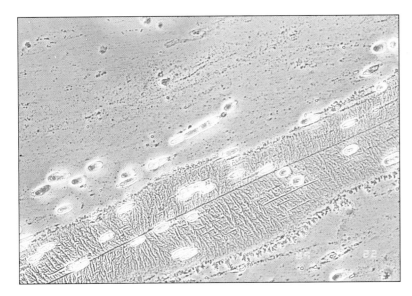

FIGURE 8-4 Microscopy of normal cervical mucus. The mucus reveals few inflammatory cells and a ferning pattern due to an increased concentration of sodium chloride during the first half of the menstrual cycle. (Original magnification, × 400.) (*Courtesy of* R. Bump, MD.)

ETIOLOGY OF CERVICITIS

Mucopurulent endocervicitis: Clinical diagnosis

Yellow or green endocervical exudate (Gram stain reveals ≥ 30
  neutrophils/high-power field)
Edema
Erythema of the zone of ectopy
Easily induced endocervical bleeding

FIGURE 8-5 Mucopurulent endocervicitis. Infection of the endocervix results in swelling and erythema of the zone of ectopy associated with friability and a yellow or a green endocervical exudate.
When Gram-stained and examined microscopically, the exudate
reveals > 30 neutrophils per high-power field [3].

Ectocervicitis: Definition and clinical variants

Definition: Inflammation of the squamous epithelium contiguous with the vagina

Clinical variants   Ulcerations or necrotic lesions (Herpes simplex virus)
                    Colpitis macularis (*Trichomonas vaginalis*)
                    Erythema with adherent vaginal secretions (*Candida albicans*)

FIGURE 8-6 Definition and clinical
variants of ectocervicitis. The squamous
epithelium of the cervix is contiguous with
the vagina. The etiology of ectocervicitis,
not surprisingly, is related to microorganisms that commonly cause a vaginitis,
ie, *Trichomonas vaginalis* and *Candida
albicans*. Herpes simplex virus can infect
both squamous and columnar epithelium.

Etiology of cervicitis

Mucopurulent endocervicitis   Idiopathic
  Chlamydia trachomatis   Ectocervicitis
  Neisseria gonorrhoeae   Herpes simplex virus
  Herpes simplex virus   *Trichomonas vaginalis*
  Cytomegalovirus   *Candida albicans*

FIGURE 8-7 Etiology of cervicitis. The presence of a purulent
exudate in the endocervical os has been highly associated with
cervical infection with *Chlamydia trachomatis*, *Neisseria gonorrhoeae*, herpes simplex virus, and cytomegalovirus. Infection with
Trichomonas vaginalis was correlated with colpitis macularis, and
inflammatory lesion of the ectocervix. Herpes simplex virus infection is correlated with ulcerative or necrotic lesions. Not infrequently, patients with mucopurulent endocervicitis or ectocervicitis will be seen in the absence of these pathogens, implying that
additional, as-yet-unrecognized causes exist.

Epidemiology of *Chlamydia trachomatis* cervicitis

Prevalence   8%–40% depending on population
                                  screened
Demographic risk factors   Young age
                                Unmarried status
                                  Lower socioeconomic conditions
Anatomic risk factor   Ectopy
Behavioral risk factor   Number of sexual partners
Microbiologic risk factor   Concurrent gonococcal infection
Hormonal risk factor   Oral contraceptive use

FIGURE 8-8 Epidemiology of *Chlamydia trachomatis* cervicitis. The
prevalence of genital *Chlamydia* infection ranges from 8% to 40%
depending on the population screened. Women traditionally noted
to be at risk for sexually transmitted diseases by virtue of their
young age, unmarried status, and living in lower socioeconomic
conditions are also at risk for *Chlamydia* infection. In addition,
cervical ectopy, in some cases induced by the use of an oral
contraceptive, appears to increase the susceptibility of young
women to *Chlamydia* infection. Moreover, new evidence suggests
that concurrent gonococcal infection may reactivate a latent
chlamydial infection [4,5].

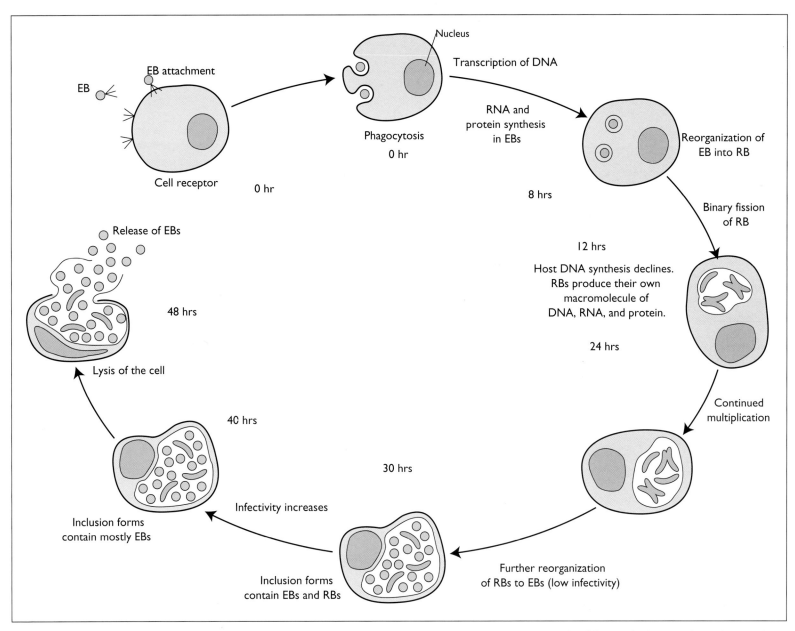

FIGURE 8-9 Life cycle of *Chlamydia trachomatis*. This obligate intracellular parasite is a common cause of mucopurulent endocer- vicitis. (EB—elementary body; RB—reticulate body.) (*Adapted from* Thompson and Washington [6].)

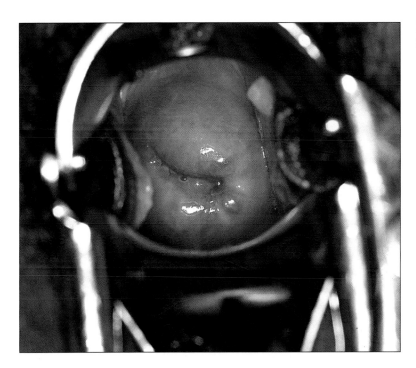

FIGURE 8-10 Cervix showing purulent endocervical discharge in chlamydial endocervicitis.

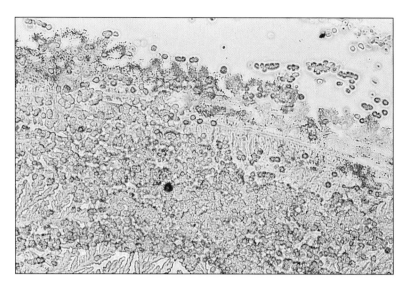

FIGURE 8-11 Microscopic examination of cervical mucus from a patient with mucopurulent endocervicitis. The mucus reveals an overabundance of inflammatory cells obliterating the background ferning pattern. (Original magnification, × 400.) (*Courtesy of* R. Bump, MD.)

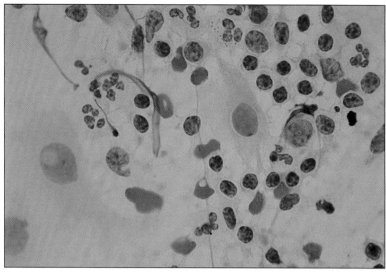

FIGURE 8-12 Papanicolaou smear from a patient with mucopurulent endocervicitis revealing an abundance of inflammatory cells.

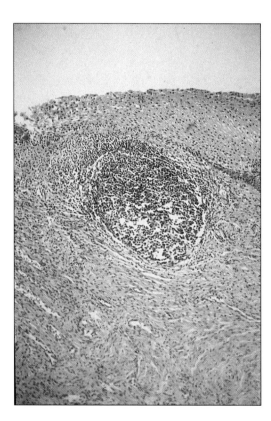

FIGURE 8-13 Cervical biopsy confirming the presence of follicular cervicitis. (*Courtesy of* J. Stasny, MD.)

Diagnosis of *Chlamydia trachomatis* cervicitis

Clinical recognition	Diagnostic tests
Mucopurulent endocervicitis	Culture
Acute urethral syndrome	Antigen detection tests
Pelvic inflammatory disease	DNA hybridization methods
Perihepatitis	Ligase chain reaction
	Polymerase chain reaction

FIGURE 8-14 Methods of diagnosis of *Chlamydia trachomatis* cervicitis. The presumptive diagnosis of chlamydial infection is difficult, but several clinical syndromes in women have been associated with this infection. Isolation of this obligate intracellular parasite requires cell culture techniques, prompting the development of more user-friendly antigen detection tests. Recent advance in highly sensitive and specific DNA amplification techniques, particularly ligase chain reaction, may lead to screening urine specimens and obviate the need for an internal examination.

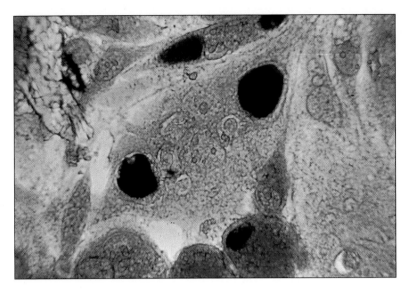

FIGURE 8-15 Culture of chlamydiae showing inclusion bodies. Isolation of *Chlamydia trachomatis* by cell culture techniques results in inclusion bodies, noted here in a McCoy cell monolayer stained with iodine. (*From* Pastorek [7]; with permission.)

Chlamydial infections: Screening criteria

Age < 25 years
New sexual partner within the past year
Suspicion of mucopurulent endocervicitis
    Suspicious discharge
    Cervical friability
Intermenstrual bleeding
No or nonbarrier contraception

FIGURE 8-16 Screening criteria for chlamydial infections. It is important to identify unrecognized chlamydial infections by appropriate screening of high-risk groups. Screening becomes cost-effective in any population in which the prevalence of infections exceeds 6%.

Chlamydial infections: Methods of screening

Test	Sensitivity, %	Specificity, %	Cost, $
Culture	65–85	100	84
Enzyme-linked immunosorbent assay	80–90	97–99	42
Monoclonal antibodies	70–89	98	45
Nucleic acid hybridization	75–96	97–99	49
Polymerase chain reaction	96	100	84
Ligase chain reaction	94	99.9	NA

NA—not applicable.

FIGURE 8-17 Methods of screening for chlamydial infections. Tests used for screening should be user-friendly so that rigorous handling of the specimen, once obtained, is not necessary. Antigen detection tests and DNA hybridization tests are currently available for such screening. Polymerase chain reaction, although available, is too expensive to recommend for use in widespread screening. Ligase chain reaction is not yet commercially available.

GONOCOCCAL CERVICITIS

Risk groups for gonococcal infections

Age 15–29 years	Early-onset sexual activity
Poor socioeconomic status	History of gonorrhea
Minority group, esp. black	Illicit drug use
Unmarried	Prostitution
Urban dweller	Multiple sex partners

FIGURE 8-18 Risk groups for gonococcal infections. Young minority women living in the inner city, where they abuse drugs and have multiple sex partners, are at high risk for contracting gonococcal infection.

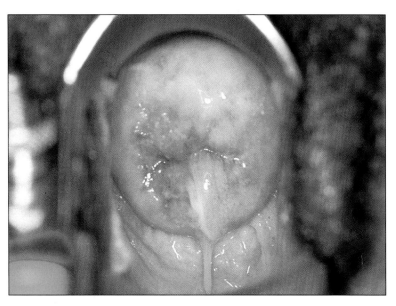

FIGURE 8-19 Mucopurulent endocervical discharge in gonococcal endocervicitis. Note the thick, yellow exudate escaping from the endocervical canal.

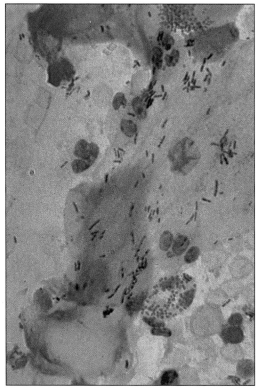

FIGURE 8-20 Gram stain of the cervical mucus revealing an inflammatory cell with intracellular gram-negative diplococci, leading to the presumptive diagnosis of gonococcal cervicitis. (*From* Handsfield [8]; with permission.)

Diagnosis of gonococcal cervicitis

Clinical recognition
  Mucopurulent endocervicitis
  Urethritis
  Pharyngitis
  Pelvic inflammatory disease
  Perihepatitis
Diagnostic tests
  Culture ("gold standard")
  DNA hybridization

FIGURE 8-21 Diagnosis of gonococcal cervicitis. Clinical recognition of syndromes associated with gonococcal infection should prompt antimicrobial therapy to cover this possibility. Culture, utilizing a modified Thayer-Martin or similar media, remains an inexpensive way of confirming the diagnosis. Utilization of DNA hybridization techniques now allows the clinician to submit one specimen to the laboratory for the detection of both *Chlamydia* and *Neisseria gonorrhoeae*.

Screening criteria for gonococcal infection

Age < 30 years
Black women
Inner city
Multiple sex partners
Prostitution
Illicit drug use
Trichomonas vaginitis

FIGURE 8-22 Screening criteria for gonococcal infection. The highest rates of gonorrhea occur in young black women living in the inner city, where they may abuse drugs or work as prostitutes. Women with *Trichomonas* vaginitis commonly have a coinfection with *Neisseria gonorrhoeae*.

Concurrent infection with *Neisseria* and *Chlamydia*

Up to 60% have coinfection with *Chlamydia*
Gonorrhea may reactivate latent chlamydial infection
Gonorrhea increases shedding of *Chlamydia* from endocervix

FIGURE 8-23 Concurrent infection with *Neisseria* and *Chlamydia*. Women with gonorrhea have the highest prevalence of chlamydial infection of any risk group, possibly due to reactivation of a latent infection [5].

OTHER BACTERIAL ENDOCERVICITIS

Bacterial vaginosis and cervicitis

Numerous studies have shown an association of BV with
  cervicitis
Up to 50% of women attending sexually transmitted disease
  clinics with mucopurulent endocervicitis have BV
Persistence of cervicitis less likely if concurrent BV is treated

BV—bacterial vaginosis.

FIGURE 8-24 Bacterial vaginosis and cervicitis. The etiology of mucopurulent endocervicitis is not readily apparent in as many as 50% of cases. Bacterial vaginosis, with its concurrent increase in concentration of potential pathogens, *eg*, anaerobes and mycoplasmas, may play a role.

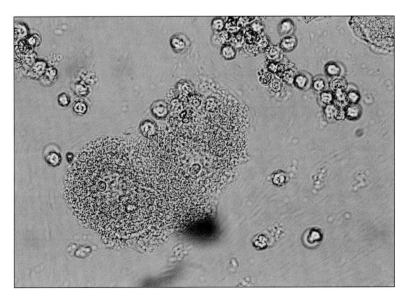

FIGURE 8-25 Microscopy of a wet mount of vaginal secretions revealing clue cells and inflammatory cells. Bacterial vaginosis is a common finding in women with concurrent cervicitis or pelvic inflammatory disease.

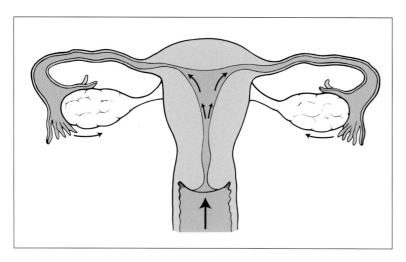

FIGURE 8-26 Pathways of ascending genital infection. Ascending spread of microorganisms can infect the endometrium and fallopian tubes causing pelvic inflammatory disease.

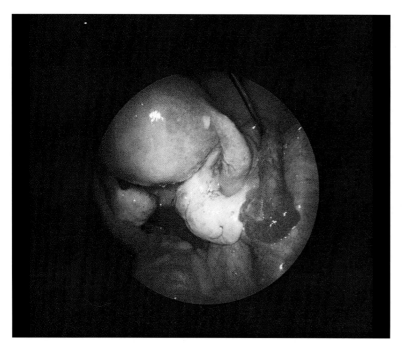

FIGURE 8-27 Laparoscopic confirmation of mild salpingitis. Laparoscopy reveals an edematous and erythematous right fallopian tube with sticky exudate apparent on the fimbria.

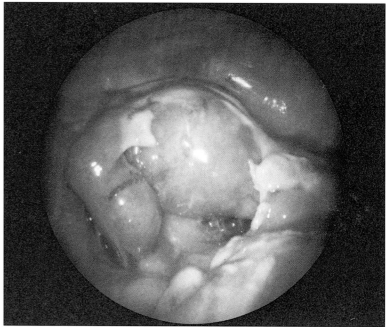

FIGURE 8-28 Laparoscopic confirmation of moderate salpingitis. Laparoscopy reveals patchy fibrin deposits on the serosal surfaces of the fallopian tubes.

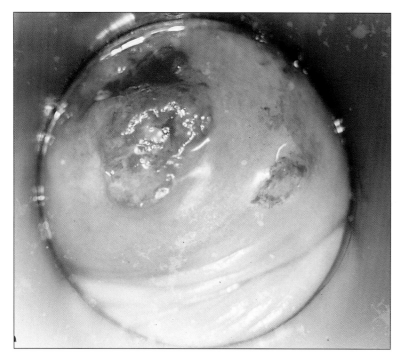

FIGURE 8-29 Tuberculosis of the cervix. Infection of the genital tract with *Mycobacterium tuberculosis* is uncommon. Although usually asymptomatic, infection usually involves the endometrium and fallopian tubes, which can lead to infertility and abnormal uterine bleeding. This figure shows a granulomatous lesion on the posterior lip of the cervix. (*Courtesy of* O. Williamson, MD.)

VIRAL CERVICITIS

Herpes Simplex Cervicitis

Herpetic cervicitis: Epidemiology

Commonly associated with first-episode, primary disease
  Isolation rate = 80%
Uncommon with recurrent vulvar lesions
  Isolation rate = 4.9%
Rare in absence of genital lesions
  Isolation rate = 0.7%

FIGURE 8-30 Epidemiology of herpetic cervicitis.

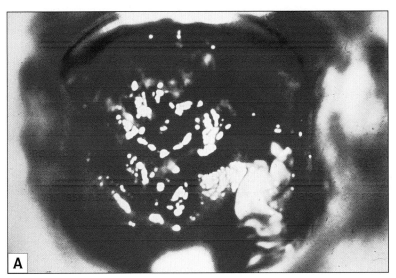

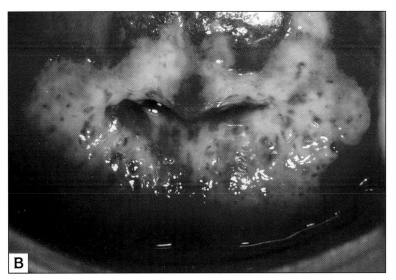

FIGURE 8-31 Gross appearance of herpes cervicitis. **A.** Primary herpes cervicitis may be associated with severe necrosis reminiscent of a cervical cancer. This appearance may precede the finding of vulvar lesions. **B.** Primary herpes cervicitis may also be characterized by increased surface vascularity and microulcerations without necrotic areas. (Panel 31A *courtesy of* Centers for Disease Control and Prevention; panel 31B *courtesy of* P. Wolner-Hanssen, MD.)

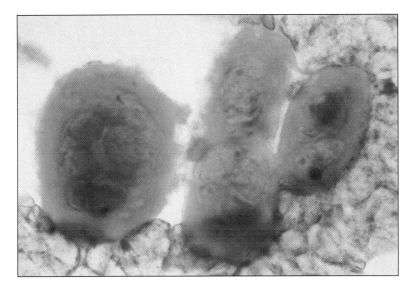

FIGURE 8-32 Papanicolaou smear from a patient with herpetic cervicitis revealing multinucleated giant cells. (*Courtesy of* J. Stasny, MD.)

Diagnosis of herpes cervicitis

Clinical recognition
  Surface ulcerations with or without necrotic areas
  Associated with primary, first-episode genital herpes
Laboratory tests
  Culture
  Rapid detection tests
    Papanicolaou stain
    Tzanck test
    Fluorescein-conjugated monoclonal antibodies
  Serologic assays

FIGURE 8-33 Diagnosis of herpes cervicitis. Genital herpes infections are commonly asymptomatic. Culture remains the "gold standard" for the confirmation of herpetic genital lesions; however, newly developed type-specific serologic methods are the most sensitive way of confirming symptomatic reactivations [9].

Complications of herpes cervicitis

Local extension
  Extragenital lesions
    Eye
    Finger
    Lip
    Buttock, groin
    Breast
  Direct extension
    Pelvic inflammatory disease
    Pelvic cellulitis
    Suppurative lymphadenitis
  Fungal superinfection

Extragenital sites
  Central nervous system complications
    Aseptic meningitis
    Sacral radiculopathy
      Urinary retention
      Constipation
      Sacral paresthesias

FIGURE 8-34 Complications of herpes cervicitis. The complications of genital herpes are related both to local extension and to spread of the virus to extragenital sites. Symptoms related to sacral radiculopathy, such as urinary retention, and fungal superinfection of the vulva are the most frequently encountered complications. (*Adapted from* Holmes [3].)

Cytomegalovirus

Epidemiology of cytomegalovirus cervicitis

Usually asymptomatic infection
Accounts for 5%–8% of cases of cervicitis

FIGURE 8-35 Epidemiology of cytomegalovirus (CMV) cervicitis. CMV infection of the cervix has been associated with cervicitis in both a sexually transmitted diseases clinic and college student population. At this point, it is unclear whether the increased detection of CMV shedding with cervicitis represents a cause or an effect of cervicitis.

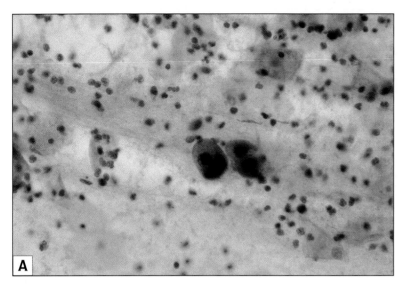

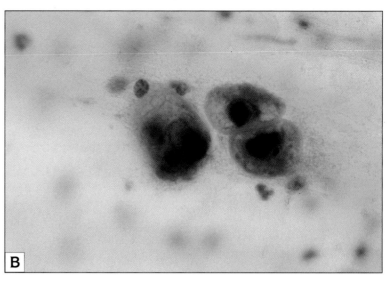

FIGURE 8-36 Papanicolaou smear in cytomegalovirus cervicitis. **A** and **B**, Papanicolaou smears show a multinucleated giant cell with background inflammatory cells consistent with cytomegalo-virus cervicitis. (Original magnification, *panel 36A*, × 40; *panel 36B*, × 100.) (*Courtesy of* J. Stasny, MD.)

Diagnosis of cytomegalovirus cervicitis

Clinical recognition
  Mucopurulent endocervicitis
Diagnostic tests
  Cell culture
  Immunocytochemical stain
  Polymerase chain reaction

FIGURE 8-37 Diagnosis of cytomegalovirus cervicitis. Cell culture remains the "gold standard" for the diagnosis of cervical cytomega-lovirus infection. Immunocytochemical stains and polymerase chain reaction can be used on biopsy specimens to confirm infection.

Human Papillomavirus

Epidemiology of HPV cervical disease

Number of physician-patient consultations increased ninefold
  between 1966 and 1987
First visits for genital warts increased tenfold over the
  same period
Evidence of HPV found on 1%–3% of all Papanicolaou smears
HPV-DNA sequences detected in almost half of sexually active
  college-aged women
Colposcopic evidence of HPV present in 25%–30% of sexually
  transmitted disease clinic patients

HPV—human papillomavirus.

FIGURE 8-38 Epidemiology of human papillomavirus cervical disease. Human papillomavirus infection may be the most common sexually transmitted disease in women.

Gynecologic lesions associated with HPV

HPV type	Lesion
6 a–f	Condylomata acuminata
	CIN I, II, III
	VIN I, II, III
11 a,b	Condylomata acuminata
	CIN I, II, III
16	Condylomata acuminata
	CIN I, II, III
	VIN I, II, III
	Bowenoid papulosis
	Carcinoma of the cervix
18	Carcinoma of the cervix
33	Bowenoid papulosis
	CIN
	Carcinoma of the cervix
34	Bowenoid papulosis
31,35,39,45,51	CIN
	Carcinoma of the cervix
30,40,42,43,44,56	CIN

CIN—cervical intraepithelial neoplasia; HPV—human
papillomavirus; VIN—vulvar intraepithelial neoplasia.

FIGURE 8-39 Gynecologic lesions associated with specific human
papillomavirus types. (*Adapted from* de Villiers [10].)

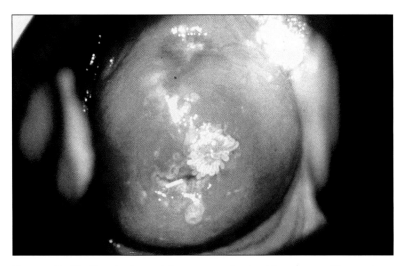

FIGURE 8-40 Cervical condyloma acuminata. Human papillomavirus
infection is a diffuse infection of the lower genital tract. Note the
condylomata on the cervix and in the vaginal fornix. (*From* American College of Obstetrics and Gynecology [1]; with permission.)

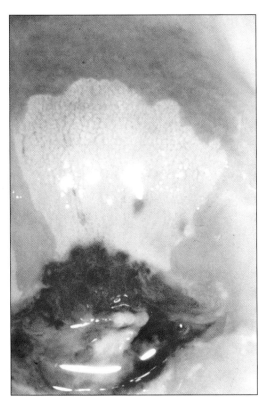

FIGURE 8-41
Acetowhitening of
cervical epithelium
showing flat condy-
loma. Application
of 3% acetic acid to
the cervix causes an
acetowhitening of
the cervical epithe-
lium, indicating the
presence of human
papillomavirus
infection (flat
condyloma).
(*Courtesy of*
H. Krebs, MD.)

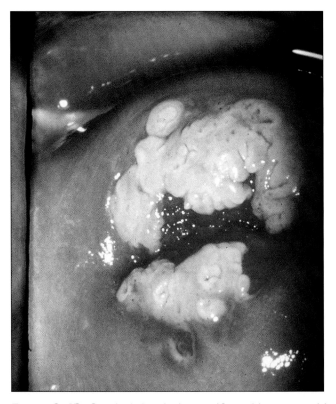

FIGURE 8-42 Cervical dysplasia manifested by acetowhitening of
the squamous epithelium. Advanced degrees of dysplasia are associated with surface vascular changes described as punctation and
mosaicism, as shown in the figure. (*Courtesy of* H. Krebs, MD.)

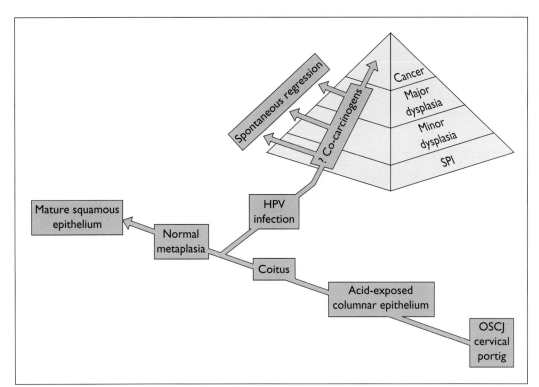

FIGURE 8-43 Progress of squamous metaplasia in the transformation zone. The process of squamous metaplasia leads to the formation of the transformation zone. Carcinogens, including human papillomavirus (HPV), acting at the squamocolumnar junction result in the dysplastic transformation of the cervical epithelial cells. (OSCJ—original squamocolumnar junction; SPI—subclinical papillomavirus infection.) (*Adapted from* Reid *et al.* [11].)

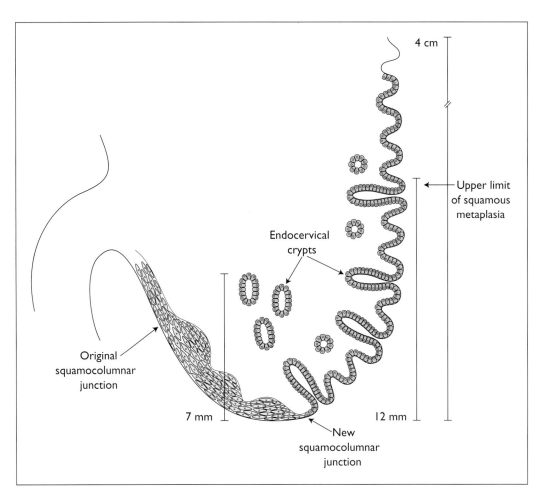

FIGURE 8-44 Anatomy of the transformation zone. The proximal migration of squamous metaplasia disguises the original squamocolumnar junction. The proximal border of the transformation zone is the upper limit of squamous metaplasia (the point at which immature squamous metaplasia abuts a circumferential ring of unaltered columnar epithelium). (*Adapted from* Reid [12].)

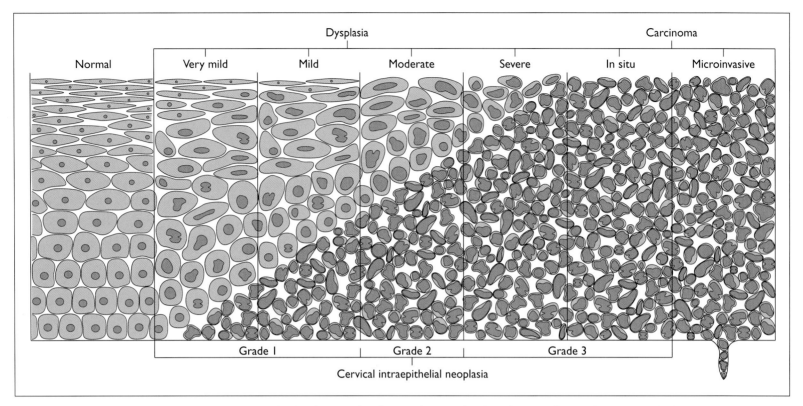

FIGURE 8-45 Depth of dysplastic involvement indicating grade of dysplasia. The depth of involvement of the cervical epithelium with dysplastic cells as reflected in a cervical biopsy determines the grade of dysplasia.

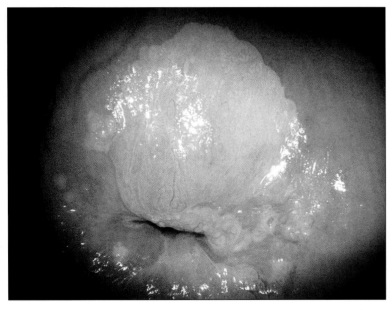

FIGURE 8-46 A large acetowhite lesion on the anterior cervix lip compatible with cervical intraepithelial neoplasia grade III. (*Courtesy of* H. Krebs, MD.)

Diagnostic methods in HPV cervicitis

Inspection
Colposcopy
Cytology/histology
Electron microscopy
Immunoperoxidase stain
Nucleic acid hybridization
Polymerase chain reaction

FIGURE 8-47 Diagnostic methods in human papillomavirus (HPV) cervicitis. HPV infection is commonly detected by gross visual inspection of a genital wart. Cytologic screening results in a large number of women being diagnosed with HPV infection by colposcopically directed biopsy. Nucleic acid hybridization techniques for screening and typing have not been embraced clinically due to their low sensitivity. Reliable serologic tests and culture techniques are not available at this time.

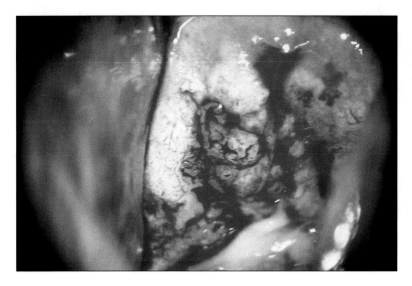

FIGURE 8-48 Squamous cell carcinoma resulting from human papillomavirus (HPV) cervicitis. The most severe complication of HPV cervicitis is squamous cell carcinoma of the cervix. Carcinoma of the cervix is related to HPV types 16 and 18. (*From* American Society for Colposcopy and Cervical Pathology [13]; with permission.)

HIV

Role of cervicitis and cervical ulceration in HIV transmission: Biologic mechanisms

Disruption of normal epithelial barriers
  (macro- or microulcerations)
Recruitment of HIV-infected cells to area of transmission
Recruitment of HIV-susceptible cells to area of transmission

FIGURE 8-49 Biologic mechanisms in the role of cervicitis and cervical ulceration in HIV transmission.

Risk estimates for HIV infection associated with classic sexually transmitted diseases

Disease	Odds ratio
Genital ulcers	3.3–18.2
Syphilis	1.8–9.9
Herpes	1.9–8.5
Gonorrhea	3.8–8.9
Genital warts	3.1–4.1
Trichomoniasis	2.3

FIGURE 8-50 Risk estimates for HIV infection associated with classic sexually transmitted diseases (STDs). Numerous observational epidemiologic studies have described an association between HIV infection and the classic STDs, *ie,* syphilis, chancroid, herpes, chlamydial infection, trichomoniasis, gonorrhea, and human papillomavirus, as well as the STD syndromes of genital ulcer disease, urethritis, and vaginal discharge.

TRICHOMONAL CERVICITIS

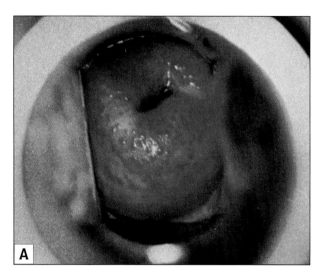 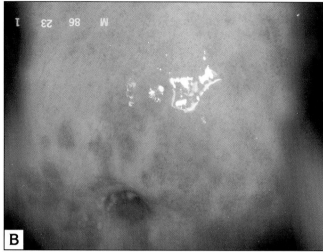

FIGURE 8-51 Colpitis macularis in trichomoniasis. **A,** A high concentration of trichomonads in the vagina cause epithelial inflammation of both the vagina and ectocervix. Cervical petechiae give the cervix a "strawberry" look in this case. **B,** A magnified view of the cervix in a patient with trichomonas vaginitis shows petechiae on the ectocervix. (Panel 51A *courtesy of* Centers for Disease Control and Prevention; panel 51B *from* Wolner-Hanssen [14]; with permission.)

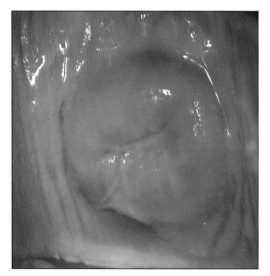 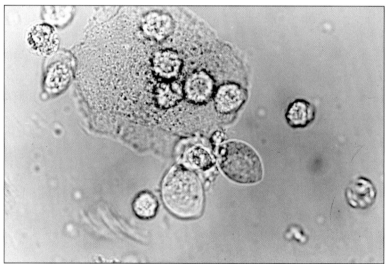

FIGURE 8-52 *Trichomonas* vaginitis causing ectocervicitis. This patient with *Trichomonas* vaginitis shows evidence of both vaginitis and ectocervicitis from her infection.

FIGURE 8-53 Microscopic examination of the vaginal secretions revealing motile trichomonads from a patient with *Trichomonas* vaginitis. (*Courtesy of* Syntex.)

MANAGEMENT OF CERVICITIS

A. Treatment of gonococcal infections

Recommended regimens
  Ceftriaxone 125 mg in single dose
    or
  Cefixime 400 mg orally in single dose
    or
  Ciprofloxacin 500 mg orally in single dose
    or
  Ofloxacin 400 mg orally in single dose
    plus
  Treatment against possible coinfections with
    Chlamydia trachomatis
  Doxycycline 100 mg orally twice a day for 7 days
    or
  Azithromycin 1 g orally in single dose

B. Treatment of chlamydial infections

Recommended regimens
  Doxycycline 100 mg orally twice a day × 7 days
    or
  Azithromycin 1 g orally in single dose

Alternative regimens
  Ofloxacin 300 mg orally twice a day × 7 days
  Erythromycin base 500 mg orally four times a day × 7 days
  Erythromycin ethylsuccinate 800 mg orally four times a day
    × 7 days
  Sulfisoxazole 500 mg orally four times a day × 10 days
    (inferior regimen)

FIGURE 8-54 Antibiotic treatment of gonococcal and chlamydial cervicitis. **A,** The Centers for Disease Control and Prevention recommend both parenteral and oral regimens for the treatment of uncomplicated gonococcal infections. **B,** Treatment of uncomplicated chlamydial infections has been revolutionized by the introduction of single-dose therapy with azithromycin [15].

Clinical follow-up of Papanicolaou smear reporting inflammatory cells ± atypia

If Papanicolaou smear shows atypical squamous cells of
  undetermined significance, with or without associated
  inflammation
Repeat Papanicolaou smear in 4–6 months
If atypia persists—perform colposcopy
If atypia resolves—repeat Papanicolaou smear in another
  4 months
If atypia returns—perform colposcopy
If atypia resolved—return to annual screening

FIGURE 8-55 Clinical follow-up of Papanicolaou smear reporting inflammatory cells with or without atypia. The Bethesda System for reporting cervical cytologic diagnosis notes that smears showing atypical squamous cells of undetermined significance (ASCUS) be considered a differential diagnosis between a benign change in reaction to a stimulus and low-grade squamous intraepithelial lesion. For this reason, women with a Papanicolaou smear showing ASCUS should have their smears repeated. Persistence of an ASCUS smear should prompt colposcopy.

Treatment of primary herpetic cervicitis

Acyclovir	200 mg orally five times a day for 7–10 days
or	
Acyclovir	400 mg orally three times a day for 7–10 days
or	
Valacyclovir	500 mg orally twice a day for 7–10 days

FIGURE 8-56 Treatment of primary herpetic cervicitis. Primary herpetic cervicitis is usually associated with severe vulvar disease and warrants therapy with one of the regimens shown. Recurrent herpetic cervicitis is inevitably asymptomatic and therefore usually not recognized in time for treatment.

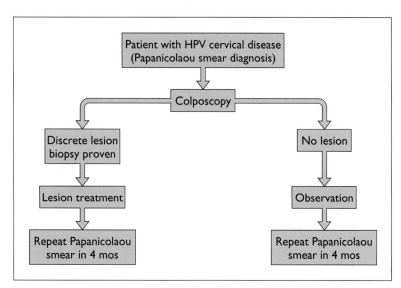

FIGURE 8-57 Approach to the patient with human papillomavirus (HPV) cervical disease. Although it is acceptable to observe patients with low-grade squamous intraepithelial lesions, such as HPV or cervical intraepithelial neoplasia grade I, many clinicians prefer to treat women with a discrete lesion noted on colposcopy. Many patients with evidence of HPV on Papanicolaou smears (koilocytosis) will not have a visible lesion at colposcopy. These patients are excellent candidates for follow-up with repeat of the Papanicolaou smear in 4 to 6 months.

Treatment options for human papillomavirus cervical disease	
Observation	Laser
Local excision	Cold coagulation
Electrocautery	Loop electrical
Cryosurgery	excisional procedure

FIGURE 8-58 Treatment options for human papillomavirus cervical disease. Studies concerning the natural history of human papillomavirus infection of the cervix suggest that approximately 50% of patients observed for a year will have spontaneous resolution of their disease. Aggressive therapy is therefore not recommended. Many clinicians believe that treating a colposcopically detected lesion with one of the above methods is preferable.

ENDOMETRITIS

Classification of endometritis
Traditional description of acute vs chronic not accurate
Most endometrial biopsies have mixed inflammatory cell populations
Upper genital tract infection with gonorrhea or chlamydiae associated with:
≥ 1 plasma cell/120× field
plus
≥ 5 neutrophils/400× field

FIGURE 8-59 Classification of endometritis. Traditional classification of endometritis based on a predominance of either "acute" inflammatory cells (*ie*, neutrophils) or "chronic" inflammatory cells (*ie*, plasma cells) does not appear to be clinically relevant. Women presenting with acute pelvic inflammatory disease uniformly have mixed cell populations noted on their endometrial biopsies. (*Adapted from* Kiviat *et al.* [16].)

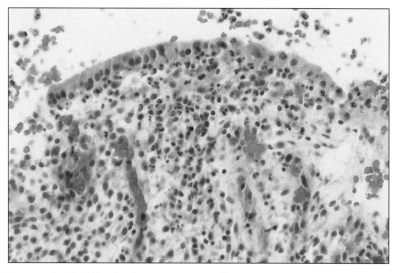

FIGURE 8-60 Histologic appearance of acute endometritis. Polymorphonuclear inflammatory cells infiltrate the surface epithelium and aggregate in the stroma of the endometrium. (Hematoxylin-eosin stain; original magnification, × 400.) (*Courtesy of* D.E. Johnson, MD.)

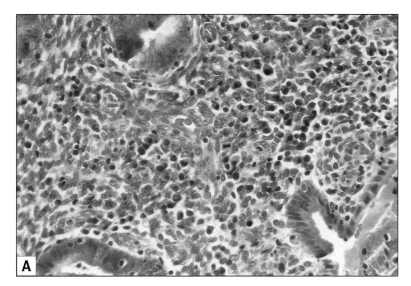

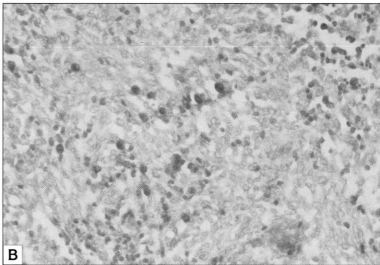

FIGURE 8-61 Histologic appearance of chronic endometritis.
A, Chronic endometritis is characterized by variable numbers of
plasma cells in the stroma. Plasma cells contain dark, eccentrically
positioned nuclei and violet cytoplasm, as shown in this hematoxylin-eosin–stained slide. **B,** A methylpyronine green stain
highlights plasma cells in cases of chronic endometritis by
staining the cytoplasm bright purple-pink, whereas the background appears pale lavender. (*Both panels,* original magnification, × 400.) (*Courtesy of* D. Johnson, MD.)

Clinical manifestations of endometritis

Symptoms	Signs
Pelvic pain	Uterine tenderness
Irregular uterine bleeding	Mucopurulent endocervicitis
Purulent vaginal discharge	Leukorrhea

FIGURE 8-62 Clinical manifestations of endometritis.

Diagnostic techniques in endometritis

Clinical recognition	Endometrial biopsy
Uterine tenderness	Pipelle™
Leukorrhea	Z-sampler™

FIGURE 8-63 Diagnostic techniques in endometritis. Inflammatory
cells are the predominant cell identified on microscopy of the vaginal
secretions. Biopsy is done with the Pipelle™ or Z-sampler™ device;
both are plastic cannulas with an internal piston to provide suction.

FIGURE 8-64 Management of endometritis.
Patients with a diagnosis of endometritis
must be assumed to have concurrent salpingitis. For this reason, treatment with one
of the recommended regimens for pelvic
inflammatory disease in an outpatient
setting is suggested [15].

Management of endometritis

Consider the diagnosis to equal PID
Patients candidates for outpatient therapy
Centers for Disease Control and Prevention recommended regimens for outpatient
  treatment of PID

Regimen A	Cefoxitin 2 g IM *plus* probenicid 1 g orally, ceftriaxone 250 mg IM,
	or cefotetan 2 g IM
	PLUS
	Doxycycline 100 mg bid × 14 days
Regimen B	Ofloxacin 400 mg orally bid
	PLUS
	Clindamycin 450 mg orally bid *or* metronidazole 500 mg bid × 14 days

bid—twice a day; IM—intramuscularly; PID—pelvic inflammatory disease.

REFERENCES

1. American College of Obstetrics and Gynecology: *Basic Colposcopy* [slide set]. Washington, DC, ACOG, 1991.

2. Critchlow CW, Wolner-Hanssen P, Eschenbach DA, *et al.*: Determinants of cervical ectopia and of cervicitis: Age, oral contraception, specific cervical infection, smoking, and douching. *Am J Obstet Gynecol* 1995, 173:534–543.

3. Holmes KK: Lower genital tract infections in women: Cystitis, urethritis, vulvovaginitis, and cervicitis. *In* Holmes KK, Mardh P-A, Sparling PF, *et al.* (eds.): *Sexually Transmitted Diseases*, 2nd ed. New York: McGraw-Hill; 1990.

4. Cates W, Wasserheit JN: Genital chlamydial infections: Epidemiology and reproductive sequelae. *Am J Obstet Gynecol* 1991, 164:1771–1781.

5. Batteiger BE, Fraiz J, Newhall WJ, *et al.*: Association of recurrent chlamydial infection with gonorrhea. *J Infect Dis* 1989, 159:661–669.

6. Thompson SE, Washington AE: Epidemiology of sexually transmitted *Chlamydia trachomatis* infections. *Epidemiol Rev* 1983, 5:96–123.

7. Pastorek EG: *Obstetrics and Gynecologic Infectious Disease*. New York: Raven Press; 1994.

8. Handsfield HH: *Color Atlas and Synopsis of Sexually Transmitted Diseases*. New York: McGraw-Hill; 1992:148.

9. Wald A, Zeh J, Selke S, *et al.*: Virologic characteristics of subclinical and symptomatic genital herpes infections. *N Engl J Med* 1995, 333:770–775.

10. de Villiers EM: Heterogeneity of the human papillomavirus group. *J Virol* 1989, 63:4898.

11. Reid R, Fu YS, Herschman BR, *et al.*: Genital warts and cervical cancer: VI. The relationship between aneuploid and polyploid cervical lesions. *Am J Obstet Gynecol* 1984, 150:189.

12. Reid R: Physical and surgical principles governing expertise with the carbon dioxide laser. *Obstet Gynecol Clin North Am* 1987, 14:526.

13. American Society for Colposcopy and Cervical Pathology: *Home Study Course, Spring 1995*. Washington, DC: ASCCP; 1995.

14. Wolner-Hanssen P: Clinical manifestations of vaginal trichomoniasis. *In* Holmes KK, Mardh P-A, Sparling PF, *et al.* (eds.): *Sexually Transmitted Diseases*, 2nd ed. New York: McGraw-Hill; 1990: Plate 20.

15. Centers for Disease Control and Prevention: 1993 Sexually transmitted diseases treatment guidelines. *MMWR* 1993, 42(RR-14):1–46.

16. Kiviat NB, Paavonen JA, Wolner-Hanssen P, *et al.*: Histopathology of endocervical infection caused by *Chlamydia trachomatis*, herpes simplex virus, *Trichomonas vaginalis*, and *Neisseria gonorrhoeae*. *Hum Pathol* 1990, 21:831–837.

SELECTED BIBLIOGRAPHY

Cates W, Wasserheit JN: Genital chlamydial infections: Epidemiology and reproductive sequelae. *Am J Obstet Gynecol* 1991, 164:1771–1781.

Critchlow CW, Wolner-Hanssen P, Eschenbach DA, *et al.*: Determinants of cervical ectopia and of cervicitis: Age, oral contraception, specific cervical infection, smoking, and douching. *Am J Obstet Gynecol* 1995, 173:534–543.

Holmes KK: Lower genital tract infections in women: Cystitis, urethritis, vulvovaginitis, and cervicitis. *In* Holmes KK, Mardh P-A, Sparling PF, *et al.* (eds.): *Sexually Transmitted Diseases*, 2nd ed. New York: McGraw-Hill; 1990.

Kiviat NB, Paavonen JA, Wolner-Hanssen P, *et al.*: Histopathology of endocervical infection caused by *Chlamydia trachomatis*, herpes simplex virus, *Trichomonas vaginalis*, and *Neisseria gonorrhoeae*. *Hum Pathol* 1990, 21:831–837.

Wald A, Zeh J, Selke S, *et al.*: Virologic characteristics of subclinical and symptomatic genital herpes infections. *N Engl J Med* 1995, 333:770–775.

CHAPTER 9

Septic Abortion

Paul Nyirjesy

EPIDEMIOLOGY

Definitions of abortion and septic abortion

Abortion: Any pregnancy terminating at 20 weeks' duration or less or in which the fetus weighs < 500 g

Septic abortion: An abortion that is complicated by infection

FIGURE 9-1 Definitions of abortion and septic abortion. Although the United States uses the definition of 20 weeks' gestation or a weight of < 500 g, some European countries use a weight of < 1000 g [1].

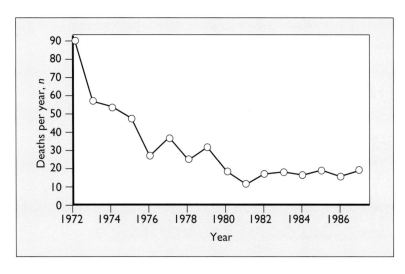

FIGURE 9-2 Number of deaths due to abortions in the United States between 1972 and 1987. Detailed statistics have been kept since 1972 about abortion-related deaths in the United States. Not only has the absolute number of deaths fallen dramatically, but so has the case–fatality rate (now at 0.4/100,000 legal induced abortions). This decrease is thought to be a reflection in the decrease in number of illegal abortions. Accurate data comparing infection rates after illegal versus legal abortion are not available. (*Adapted from* Koonin *et al.* [2].)

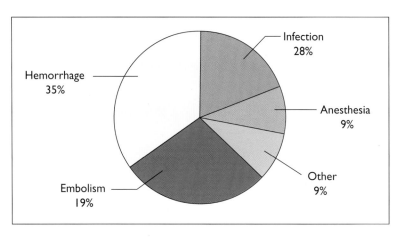

FIGURE 9-3 Causes of deaths due to abortion in the United States between 1979 and 1986. Although infection accounts for only 7.6% of total maternal deaths in the United States, it caused 28% of abortion-related deaths from 1979 to 1986. (*Adapted from* Koonin *et al.* [3].)

Infection rates following invasive uterine procedures

Procedure	Infection rate	Reference
Legal abortion	15/497	[4]
Amniocentesis	0/4606	[5]
Chorionic villus sampling	1/943	[6]
Percutaneous umbilical blood sampling	0/606	[7]

FIGURE 9-4 Infection rates following invasive uterine procedures. Infection can occur following any invasive uterine procedure. Although frank infection after procedures other than abortion is rare, published rates may underestimate the problem. Procedure-related fetal losses may be the result of occult infection [4–7].

Risk factors for postabortal infection

Age < 20 yrs
Nulliparity
Greater duration of pregnancy
Multiple sexual partners
History of pelvic inflammatory disease or gonorrhea
Current genital infection
  Bacterial vaginosis
  Chlamydial or gonococcal cervicitis

FIGURE 9-5 Risk factors for postabortal infection. Risk factors for postabortal pelvic infection have been established in several epidemiologic studies. In many ways, they resemble the risk factors for pelvic inflammatory disease in general, suggesting similarities in terms of microbial etiology and pathogenesis [8].

PATHOGENESIS AND ETIOLOGY

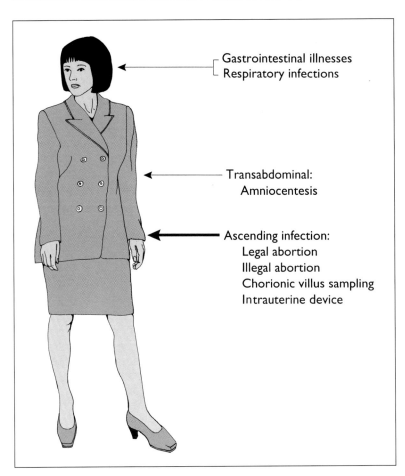

Gastrointestinal illnesses
Respiratory infections

Transabdominal:
  Amniocentesis

Ascending infection:
  Legal abortion
  Illegal abortion
  Chorionic villus sampling
  Intrauterine device

FIGURE 9-6 Pathogenesis of septic abortion. The vast majority of septic abortions occur as a result of ascending infection from the vagina, frequently with some associated traumatic event. However, cases of septic abortion in which the infecting organism was thought to be ingested (*Listeria monocytogenes, Clostridium jejuni*), inhaled (*Haemophilus influenzae*), or introduced transabdominally have been reported.

Microbial etiology of septic abortion

Aerobes	Anaerobes
Streptococcus spp	*Bacteriodes* spp
Enterococcus spp	*Prevotella* spp
Staphylococcus aureus	*Fusobacterium*
Escherichia coli	*Peptococcus* spp
Klebsiella pneumoniae	*Peptostreptococcus*
Proteus mirabilis	*Veillonella* spp
Pseudomonas aeruginosa	*Clostridium* spp
Enterobacter cloacae	
Neisseria gonorrhoeae	Other
Mycoplasma hominis	*Chlamydia trachomatis*

FIGURE 9-7 Microbial etiology of septic abortion. The microbes responsible for most septic abortions reflect the flora of the vagina, both normal and abnormal. Anaerobes frequently figure prominently among the organisms isolated from patients, especially *Bacteroides* species. *Clostridium perfringens* has been associated mainly with illegal abortions [9].

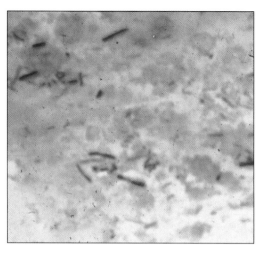

FIGURE 9-8 Gram stain of *Clostridium perfringens*. Gram stain reveals large, gram-positive rods with a "freight-car" morphology typical of *C. perfringens*. Some forms may be de-stained and appear as gram-negative. (*Courtesy of* M. Finegold, MD.)

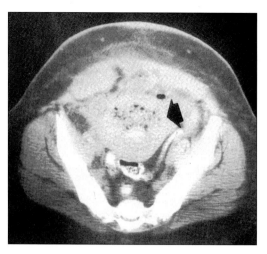

FIGURE 9-9 Computed tomography scan showing gas bubbles within enlarged uterus of a woman with postpartum uterine infection due to *Clostridium perfringens*. In contrast to anaerobic infections that may produce gas-forming abscesses in the open spaces of the abdomen or pelvic organs, *C. perfringens* may produce gas bubbles in the tissues of the soft organs. In this case of a postpartum uterine infection, gas bubbles (*arrow*) are seen extending concentrically into the myometrium. (*From* Dylewski *et al.* [10]; with permission.)

CLINICAL MANIFESTATIONS

Symptoms of septic abortion
Fever and chills
Abdominal pain
Vaginal bleeding
Passage of placental tissue

FIGURE 9-10 Symptoms of septic abortion. Fever and lower abdominal or pelvic pain are frequently the most prominent symptoms in septic abortions. The third part of the triad, bleeding, may vary from a small amount of malodorous bloody discharge to frank hemorrhage.

Signs of septic abortion
Fever, tachycardia, tachypnea, hypotension
Lower abdominal tenderness
Bloody or malodorous vaginal discharge
Cervical os may be open or closed
Uterine tenderness
Adnexal masses
Septic shock and disseminated intravascular coagulation

FIGURE 9-11 Signs of septic abortion. The signs of septic abortion are those arising as a result of bacteremia and its sequelae as well as of the local uterine infection.

Clues to clostridial sepsis
Pain out of proportion to findings
Tachycardia
"Toxic" appearance
Gram-positive rods in cervical discharge or on blood culture
Gas in soft tissues
Intravascular hemolysis

FIGURE 9-12 Although *Clostridium perfringens* infection causes only an estimated 1.7% of septic abortions, these infections are considered the most lethal. The production of various exotoxins and hyaluronidase permits early invasion and destruction of surrounding tissues, as well as hemolysis of erythrocytes and destruction of platelets. In patients with clostridial infections, early diagnosis and treatment are essential to patient survival [11].

Evaluation of the patient with suspected septic abortion

Complete blood count, prothrombin time, partial
  thromboplastin time
Electrolytes, blood urea nitrogen, creatinine
Cervical Gram stain and culture
Posteroanterior and lateral chest films
Flat and upright radiographs of abdomen and pelvis
Pelvic ultrasound

Figure 9-13 Evaluation of the patient with suspected septic abortion. Patients with septic abortion need a thorough evaluation of both the local process as well as its systemic effects. Cervical Gram stain and culture will frequently reveal an increase in polymorphonuclear leukocytes and a mixed coccobacillary flora. Blood cultures will be positive in up to 38% of patients [9].

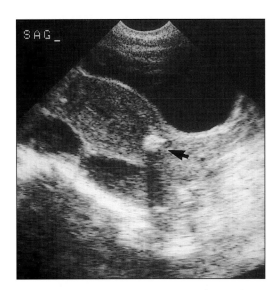

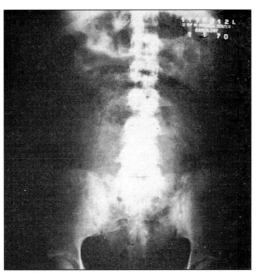

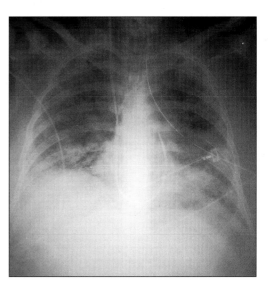

Figure 9-14 Pelvic ultrasound of a patient with septic abortion. The ultrasound reveals echogenic material near the cervical os (*arrow*) and fluid higher up in the uterine cavity.

Figure 9-15 Abdominal radiograph of patient with a postabortal *Clostridium perfringens* infection. Whereas gas beneath the diaphragm is suggestive of a bowel perforation occurring during the abortion, gas within the myometrium typically results from *C. perfringens* infection. In either situation, operative management of the patient becomes mandatory. (*From* Eaton *et al.* [11]; with permission.)

Figure 9-16 Chest radiograph of a woman with adult respiratory distress syndrome. Although adult respiratory distress syndrome may be the most prominent finding in a patient in septic shock from septic abortion, one must remember also to look underneath the diaphragm for evidence of a bowel perforation.

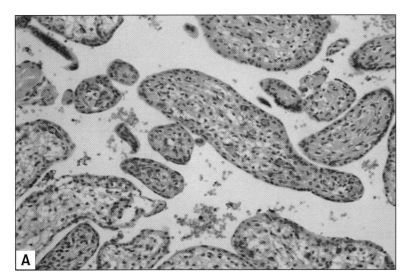

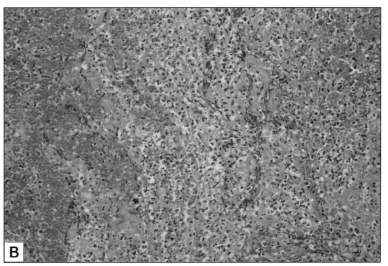

Figure 9-17 Products of conception in patients with spontaneous and septic abortions. **A,** In a patient with a spontaneous abortion, the products of conception reveal chorionic villi with a noticeable lack of inflammatory cells or necrotic debris. (× 100.) **B,** In a patient with septic abortion, the products of conception reveal amorphous necrotic debris with moderate inflammation. (× 100.)

COMPLICATIONS

A. Acute complications of septic abortion
Septic shock
Uterine gas gangrene
Bowel perforation
Tuboovarian abscess
Septic pelvic thrombophlebitis
Death

B. Chronic complications of septic abortion
Tubal infertility
Pelvic adhesions
Asherman's syndrome
Cervical incompetence

FIGURE 9-18 Complications of septic abortion. The complications of septic abortion reflect those of the acute process, as well as the sequelae of uninfected abortions (*eg*, cervical incompetence, Asherman's syndrome) and of any uterine infection (*eg*, tubal infertility, pelvic adhesions). **A**, Acute complications. **B**, Chronic complications.

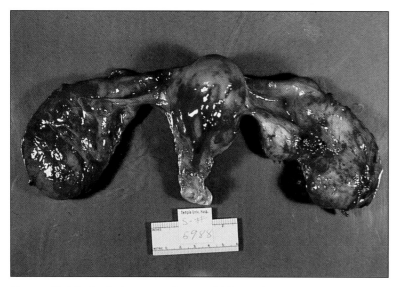

FIGURE 9-19 Pathology specimen of bilateral tuboovarian abscesses. In addition to the obvious hydrosalpinges and tuboovarian abscesses, there is fibrinous debris on the surfaces of the uterus, fallopian tubes, and ovaries.

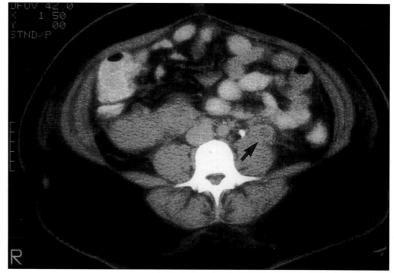

FIGURE 9-20 Computed tomography scan of a woman with septic pelvic thrombophlebitis. A filling defect is seen in the left ovarian vein (*arrow*). Frequently, the computed tomography scan will be negative, and a diagnosis must be made on the basis of excluding other causes of fever in a patient who fails to respond to appropriate therapy within 48 to 72 hours. In such women, a successful response to heparin therapy will confirm the diagnosis and treat her condition.

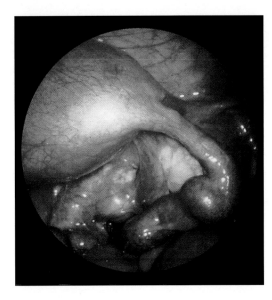
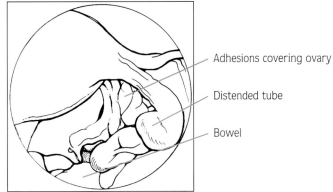

Adhesions covering ovary

Distended tube

Bowel

FIGURE 9-21 Tubal blockage following septic abortion. Infertility occurring as a result of postabortal tubal damage may present years after the precipitating infection. This laparoscopic picture demonstrates a distal blockage of the right fallopian tube, which is distended with methylene blue dye. The right ovary, covered with filmy adhesions, can be seen adjacent to the tube. (*From* Gordon and Lewis [12]; with permission.)

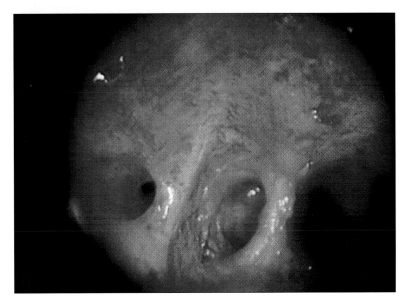

FIGURE 9-22 Hysteroscopic view of intrauterine adhesions, obliterating the upper portion of the uterine cavity. These adhesions frequently are secondary to puerperal endometrial curettage. They may lead to secondary amenorrhea (Asherman's syndrome), other menstrual irregularities, infertility, or recurrent abortion. (*From* Siegler *et al.* [13]; with permission.)

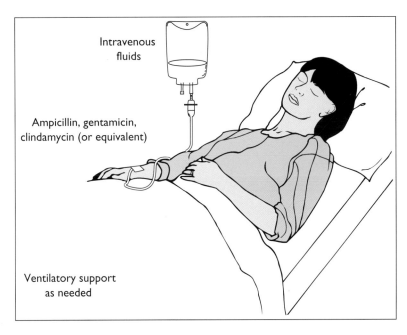

Intravenous fluids

Ampicillin, gentamicin, clindamycin (or equivalent)

Ventilatory support as needed

FIGURE 9-23 Management of the patient with septic abortion. In treating women with septic abortion, the first priority is medical stabilization with the correction of fluid and electrolyte imbalances. Antibiotic therapy must be broad and should include adequate anaerobic and gram-negative coverage. Transfusion, ventilatory support, and vasopressor support may also be necessary.

MANAGEMENT AND PREVENTION

Antibiotic selection in septic abortion

Ampicillin, gentamicin, and clindamycin
Other aminoglycosides or aztreonam may be substituted for
  gentamicin
Cefoxitin and doxycycline
Alternatives to cefoxitin include cefotetan, ticarcillin/clavu-
  lanate, ampicillin/sulbactam, piperacillin/tazobactam, and
  imipenem

FIGURE 9-24 Antibiotic selection in septic abortion. Antibiotic selection for the treatment of septic abortion is similar to that for treatment of other pelvic infections. Initial antibiotics should mainly cover the normal vaginal flora and sexually transmitted organisms such as *Neisseria gonorrhoeae* and *Chlamydia trachomatis*. Although penicillin G is generally considered the drug of choice for patients with clostridial infections, alternatives such as clindamycin, metronidazole, tetracycline, and imipenem demonstrate *in vitro* activity against most strains and sidestep concerns about growing penicillin resistance.

Surgical treatment of septic abortion

Curettage of retained products
Laparoscopy if uterine perforation suspected
Laparotomy with possible:
  Drainage or removal of abscess
  Total abdominal hysterectomy

FIGURE 9-25 Surgical treatment of septic abortion. Dilation and curettage should be performed routinely to remove any infected debris within the uterus. If uterine perforation is suspected or if the patient fails to respond to therapy, laparoscopy or laparotomy is indicated to look for hemoperitoneum, bowel perforation, or adnexal abscess. Although the exact role of hysterectomy remains controversial, it should be considered in the presence of clostridial infection, unless the patient responds rapidly to medical therapy.

Preventive measures in septic abortion

Avoidance of unwanted pregnancy
Provision of legal abortion
Prophylactic antibiotics
  Doxycycline, 100 mg before and 200 mg after procedure

FIGURE 9-26 Preventive measures in septic abortion. In countries where induced abortion is legal, morbidity and mortality from septic abortion remain rare events. Therefore, general preventive measures go well beyond simple antibiotic prophylaxis.

REFERENCES

1. Cunningham FG, MacDonald PC, Gant NF: Abortion. *In* Cunningham FG, MacDonald PC, Gant NF (eds.): *Williams Obstetrics*, 18th ed. Norwalk, CT: Appleton & Lange; 1989:489.

2. Koonin LM, Smith JC, Ramick M, Lawson HW: Abortion surveillance—United States, 1989. *MMWR* 1992, 41(SS-5):1–33.

3. Koonin LM, Atrash HK, Lawson HW, Smith JC: Maternal mortality surveillance, United States, 1979–1986. *MMWR* 1991, 40(SS-2):10.

4. Levallois P, Rioux JE: Prophylactic antibiotics for suction curettage abortion: Results of a clinical controlled trial. *Am J Obstet Gynecol* 1988, 158:100–105.

5. Daffos F, Capella-Pavlovsky M, Forestier F: Fetal blood sampling during pregnancy with use of a needle guided by ultrasound: A study of 606 consecutive cases. *Am J Obstet Gynecol* 1985, 153:655–660.

6. Tabor A, Philip J, Madsen M, *et al.*: Randomised controlled trial of genetic amniocentesis in 4606 low-risk women. *Lancet* 1986, 1:1287–1293.

7. Jackson LG, Zachary JM, Fowler SE, *et al.*: A randomized comparison of transcervical and transabdominal chorionic-villus sampling: The U.S. National Institute of Child Health and Human Development Chorionic-Villus Sampling and Amniocentesis Study Group. *N Engl J Med* 1992, 327:594–598.

8. Sawaya GF, Grimes DA: Preventing postabortal infection. *Contemp Ob/Gyn* 1994, 39:53–60.

9. Chow AW, Marshall JR, Guze LB: A double-blind comparison of clindamycin with penicillin plus chloramphenicol in treatment of septic abortion. *J Infect Dis* 1977, 135:S35–S39.

10. Dylewski J, Wiesenfeld H, Latour A: Postpartum uterine infection with *Clostridium perfringens. Rev Infect Dis* 1989, 11:470–473.

11. Eaton CJ, Peterson EP: Diagnosis and acute management of patients with advanced clostridial sepsis complicating abortion. *Am J Obstet Gynecol* 1971, 109:1162–1166.

12. Gordon AG, Lewis BV: *Gynecological Endoscopy*. Philadelphia: J.B. Lippincott; 1988:4.9.

13. Siegler AM, Valle RF, Lindenmann HJ, Mencaglia L: *Therapeutic Hysteroscopy: Indications and Techniques*. St. Louis: C.V. Mosby; 1990.

SELECTED BIBLIOGRAPHY

Atrash HK, MacKay HT, Binkin NJ, Hogue CJR: Legal abortion mortality in the United States: 1972 to 1982. *Am J Obstet Gynecol* 1987, 156:605–612.

Cunningham FG, MacDonald PC, Gant NF: Abortion. *In* Cunningham FG, MacDonald PC, Gant NF (eds.): *Williams Obstetrics*, 18th ed. Norwalk, CT: Appleton & Lange; 1989:489–509.

Grimes DA, Cates W Jr, Selik RM: Fatal septic abortion in the United States, 1975–1977. *Obstet Gynecol* 1981, 57:739–744.

Sweet RL, Gibbs RS: Postabortion infection and septic shock. *In* Sweet RL, Gibbs RS (eds.): *Infectious Disease of the Female Genital Tract*, 2nd ed. Baltimore: Williams & Wilkins; 1990:229–240.

CHAPTER 10

Tuboovarian Abscesses

Harold C. Wiesenfeld
Richard L. Sweet

PATHOGENESIS AND ETIOLOGY

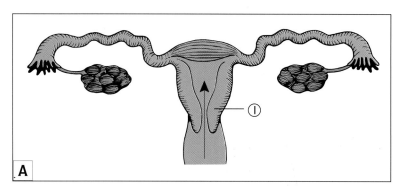

A

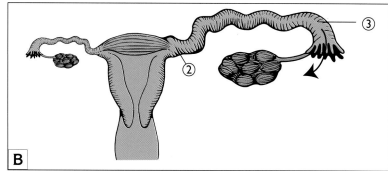

B

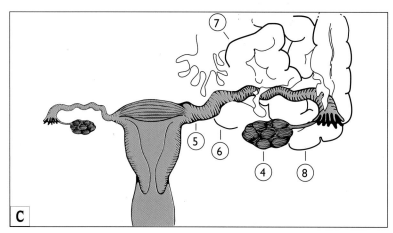

C

FIGURE 10-1 Pathogenesis of tuboovarian abscesses (TOAs). Most commonly, TOAs result from the ascent of pathogens and vaginal flora to the upper genital tract. Infection of the fallopian tube ensues, followed by spillage of purulent exudate into the peritoneal cavity. **A,** Ascent of pathogens and vaginal flora from the lower to the upper genital tract (*1*). **B,** Destruction of tubal epithelium with pyosalpinx formation (*2*). Spillage of purulent exudate from the fimbrial end into the peritoneal cavity (*3*). Damage to the capsule of the ovary (following ovulation) has been postulated to initiate ovarian involvement in the abscess formation. **C,** Formation of TOA with localization of the infectious process by contiguous structures: ovary (*4*), fallopian tube (*5*), omentum (*6*), small intestine (*7*), and large intestine (*8*).

Microbiology of tuboovarian abscesses	
Escherichia coli	37%
Bacteroides fragilis	22%
Prevotella bivia	26%
Prevotella disiens	26%
Streptococcus	—
Peptostreptococcus	19%
Neisseria gonorrhoeae	4%
Actinomyces israelii	—

FIGURE 10-2 Microbiology of tuboovarian abscesses (TOAs). Most TOAs are polymicrobial. Cultures often feature a mixture of anaerobic and aerobic organisms, commonly including *Escherichia coli* and *Bacteroides fragilis.* Although they are major etiologic agents in pelvic inflammatory disease, *Neisseria gonorrhoeae* and *Chlamydia trachomatis* are rarely recovered from abscess cavities, yet they undoubtedly play an important role in the pathogenesis of many TOAs. Additionally, α-hemolytic and group B β-hemolytic streptococci are occasionally among the organisms isolated [1].

Predisposing factors in the development of tuboovarian abscesses
Acute PID
Previous episodes of PID
Multiple sexual partners
Use of intrauterine device
No contraceptive use
Low socioeconomic status
Adolescence
PID—pelvic inflammatory disease.

FIGURE 10-3 Predisposing factors in the development of tuboovarian abscesses (TOAs). TOAs are present in up to one third of women hospitalized with acute pelvic inflammatory disease (PID). Risk factors for TOAs are similar to those for PID. Both PID and TOAs are important sequelae of sexually transmitted diseases and are frequently seen in women at risk for sexually transmitted diseases, such as adolescents and those with multiple sexual partners. TOA may reflect a subsequent stage of either clinically recognized or unrecognized PID, and as such, up to one half of patients with TOAs have a prior history of PID.

CLINICAL FEATURES

A. Clinical findings in tuboovarian abscesses: Symptoms

Abdominal/pelvic pain	> 90%
Fever and chills	50%
Vaginal discharge	28%
Nausea and vomiting	26%
Abnormal vaginal bleeding	21%

B. Clinical findings in tuboovarian abscesses: Physical and laboratory findings

Fever (60%–80% of patients)
Lower abdominal tenderness
"Signs of peritonitis" (*eg*, guarding/rebound)
Excess cervicovaginal secretions
Evidence of cervicitis
Palpation of adnexal mass
Leukocytosis (66%–80% of patients)

FIGURE 10-4 Clinical findings in tuboovarian abscess. **A**, Symptoms. **B**, Physical and laboratory findings. The clinical presentation of patients with tuboovarian abscesses is similar to that of women with acute pelvic inflammatory disease. Most women present with abdominal and/or pelvic pain. The presence of other symptoms and findings, such as fever, increased vaginal discharge, and leukocytosis may be variable. Palpation of an adnexal mass may be inadequate due to the pelvic pain and tenderness [2].

Atypical presentations of tuboovarian abscesses

Fever of unknown origin
Deep dyspareunia
Chronic lower back pain
Abnormal vaginal bleeding

FIGURE 10-5 Atypical presentations of tuboovarian abscesses (TOAs). Women with TOAs may not present with symptoms usually associated with upper genital tract infection. Because of loculation and isolation of the infectious process by contiguous structures, more subtle signs and symptoms may be present. Physical examination and selective use of diagnostic imaging procedures may help confirm the presence of TOAs.

Differential diagnosis of tuboovarian abscesses

Endometriosis (endometrioma)
Ectopic pregnancy
Appendicitis/periappendiceal abscess
Ovarian cyst/neoplasm (benign or malignant)
Pelvic hematoma
Diverticular abscess
Inflammatory bowel disease

FIGURE 10-6 Differential diagnosis of tuboovarian abscesses. The differential diagnosis of tuboovarian abscess is broad, involving several organ systems. In addition to the history and physical examination, further investigation with ultrasound or computed tomography scanning is typically warranted. As evident from the list of differential diagnoses, other surgical emergencies must be excluded.

Sequelae of tuboovarian abscesses
Early
Rupture of TOA
Pelvic thrombophlebitis/ovarian vein thrombosis
Late
Infertility
Ectopic pregnancy
Chronic pelvic pain
Recurrent pelvic inflammatory disease/TOA

TOA—tuboovarian abscess.

FIGURE 10-7 Sequelae of tuboovarian abscesses. The most serious short-term consequence of tuboovarian abscesses is rupture of the abscess. This surgical emergency has historically been associated with a high mortality rate, but the advent of surgical therapy and broad-spectrum antibiotics has reduced the mortality to < 2%. Long-term sequelae are a major health concern. Less than 20% of women are able to conceive spontaneously, and many women suffer chronic pelvic pain and subsequent episodes of pelvic infections.

Effect of tuboovarian abscesses on long-term fertility	
Study	Pregnancies achieved, % (no./women)
Reed *et al.* (1991)	8 (6/75)
Ginsburg *et al.* (1980)	9 (9/105)
Henry-Suchet* (1984)	13 (3/24)

*Women with bilateral tuboovarian abscesses.

FIGURE 10-8 Effect of tuboovarian abscesses (TOAs) on long-term fertility. Accurate information on fertility rates following TOAs is lacking, mainly due to poor compliance with follow-up, nonstandardized definitions of infertility, and the lack of prospective studies. Additionally, management of TOAs is variable. Best estimates of fertility following TOAs range from 5% to 15% [3–5].

Effect of TOAs on tubal damage: Findings on second-look laparoscopy after laparoscopic treatment of TOAs	
Normal adnexae	12 (48%)
Unilateral adhesions	5 (20%)
Bilateral adhesions with tubal obstruction	8 (32%)
Required later surgery	9 (36%)

TOA—tuboovarian abscess.

FIGURE 10-9 Effect of tuboovarian abscesses (TOAs) on tubal damage: Findings on second-look laparoscopy after laparoscopic treatment of TOAs. Most long-term sequelae from TOAs result from pelvic adhesion formation during the acute illness and the convalescent period. Tubal impairment, either due to adhesive disease or fallopian tube mucosal damage, results in tubal-factor infertility, ectopic pregnancy formation, and chronic pelvic pain. Subsequent surgical intervention is often required for patients with chronic pelvic pain, infertility, and recurrent infections. Limited data are available on tubal damage; these figures represent an unselected subset of patients undergoing a second laparoscopy following initial laparoscopic drainage of TOAs. The frequencies of sequelae may be underestimated [5].

DIAGNOSTIC PROCEDURES

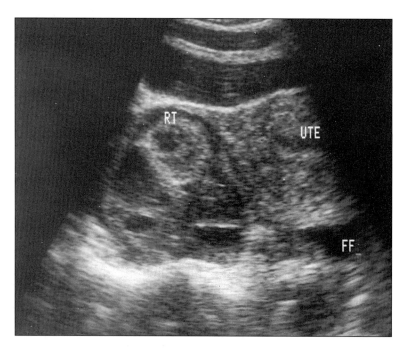

FIGURE 10-10 Ultrasound image of tuboovarian abscess. The mass in the right adnexa (RT) demonstrates a complex architecture with septations, internal echoes, and thickened walls. Free fluid (FF), which may represent a purulent exudate, is often seen. (UTE—uterus.)

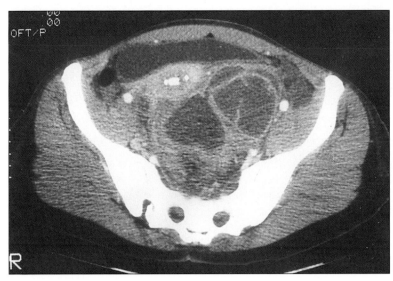

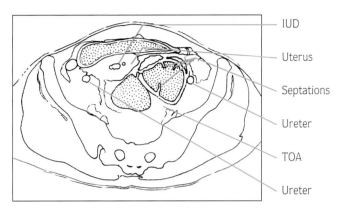

FIGURE 10-11 Computed tomography image of a large tuboovarian abscess (TOA). Internal septations and thickened walls are readily demonstrated in this inflammatory multicystic complex. There is often a loss of fat planes in the pelvis. Hydroureter is occasionally seen. The differential diagnosis includes endometrioma, diverticular and periappendiceal abscess, ovarian neoplasms (benign and malignant), and pelvic hematomas. The presence of an intrauterine device (IUD), can be seen in this image.

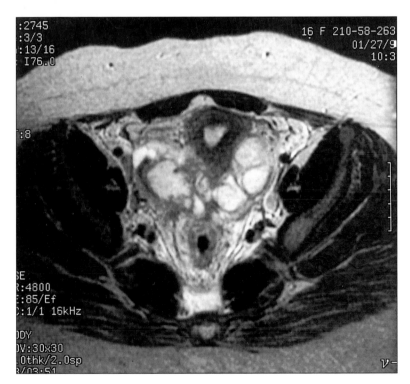

FIGURE 10-12 Magnetic resonance image of bilateral tuboovarian abscesses. Multilocular masses are clearly evident in both adnexae, extending into the posterior cul-de-sac.

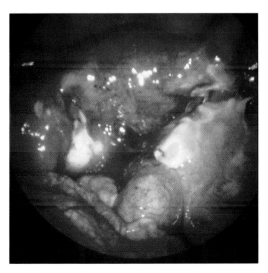

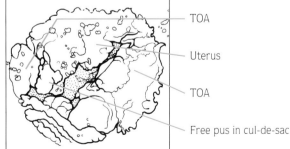

FIGURE 10-13 Laparoscopic view of bilateral tuboovarian abscesses (TOAs). Laparoscopy remains the "gold standard" for the diagnosis of pelvic inflammatory disease and TOA. Direct visualization of the pelvis in women with TOAs reveals the characteristic dilated fallopian tubes with adherent ovaries and associated pelvic and abdominal structures. Purulent exudate may be present on initial inspection or following manipulation and disruption of the pelvic adhesions. The infected tissues are extremely friable, and aggressive handling may be unwarranted.

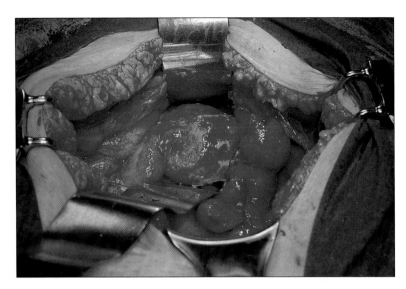

FIGURE 10-14 Intraoperative appearance of a tuboovarian abscess. Large bilateral inflammatory masses are easily seen, with hyperemia of the tissues, formation of fibrinous exudate, and multiple adhesions. Tissue planes are often very difficult to define, making dissection difficult. Return of normal bowel function in the postoperative period is delayed due to ongoing peritonitis.

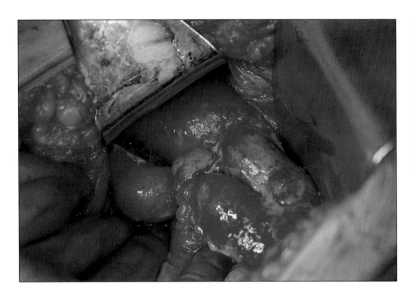

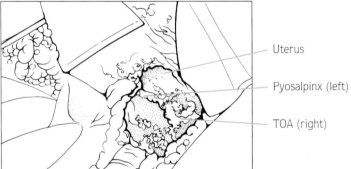

FIGURE 10-15 Operative view at laparotomy of a patient with a right-sided tuboovarian abscess (TOA) and a left pyosalpinx. Fresh adhesion formation and fibrinous exudate can be easily appreciated.

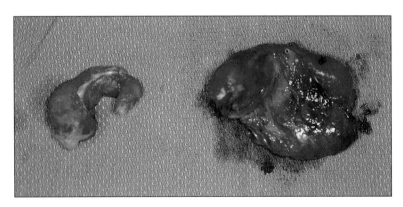

FIGURE 10-16 Photograph of resected tissue from a patient with a tuboovarian abscess. The smaller structure on the left is a distended fallopian tube characteristic of a pyosalpinx. Aspiration of the contents of this fallopian tube yielded purulent material. On the right is the adnexa, measuring 8 cm in length. In this tuboovarian complex, the distended fallopian tube is visualized above the densely adherent ovary. Tissue planes between the fallopian tube and ovary have been obliterated by the infectious process. Normal ovarian ultrastructure is not discernible due to the large inflammatory process and adhesion formation.

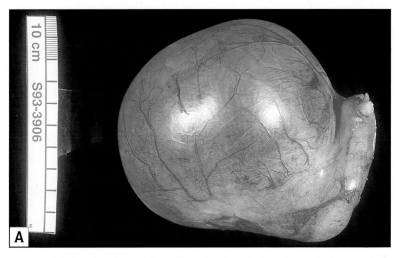

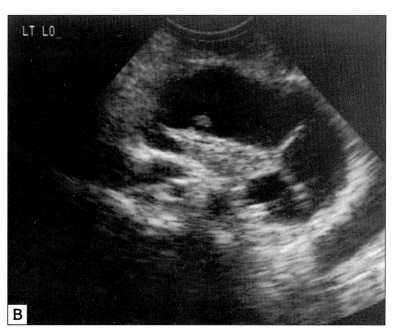

FIGURE 10-17 Hydrosalpinx. Proximal and distal tubal obstruction following salpingitis may lead to the collection of sterile watery fluid in the lumen of the fallopian tube. Hydrosalpinx may cause pelvic pain and dyspareunia or may be asymptomatic. **A**, Gross appearance of a hydrosalpinx. **B**, Ultrasound image of the fluid-filled fallopian tube.

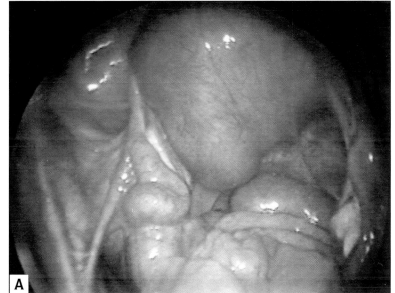

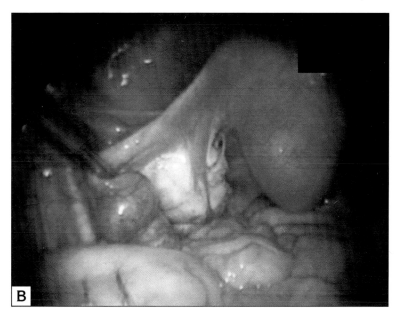

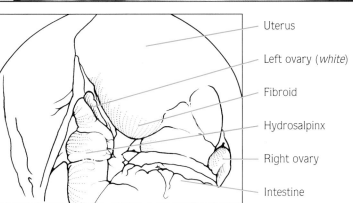

- Uterus
- Left ovary (*white*)
- Fibroid
- Hydrosalpinx
- Right ovary
- Intestine

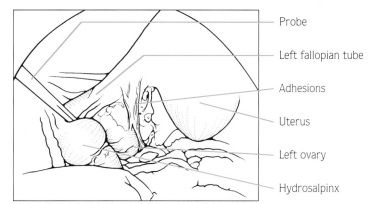

- Probe
- Left fallopian tube
- Adhesions
- Uterus
- Left ovary
- Hydrosalpinx

FIGURE 10-18 Laparoscopic view of a left-sided hydrosalpinx. **A**, This structure appears dilated and tortuous and is filled with clear fluid. **B**, When the fallopian tube is retracted, the ovary can clearly be seen distinct from the tube. The presence of adhesions from the fallopian tube to the ovary are noted, likely indicative of previous upper genital tract infection (*ie*, pelvic inflammatory disease). An incidental finding was a myoma (fibroid) in the posterior wall of the uterus.

TREATMENT

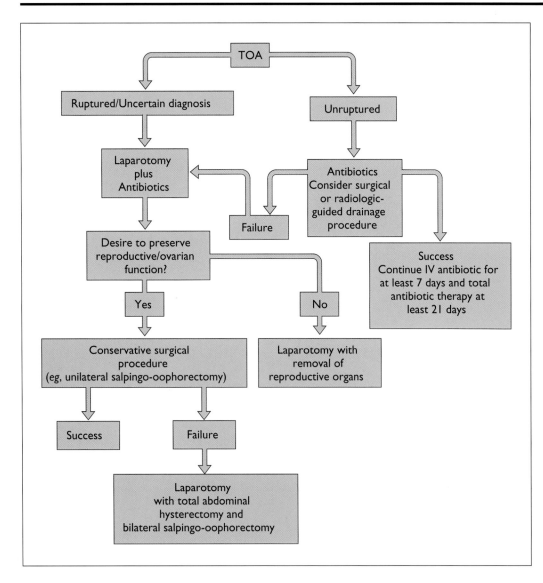

FIGURE 10-19 Approach to the management of tuboovarian abscess(TOA). Medical management utilizing broad-spectrum antimicrobials may be selected when there is certainty of diagnosis, the patient is clinically stable, and the abscess is unruptured. Otherwise, operative intervention with either conservative or definitive procedures is often necessary. Radiologic-guided drainage procedures (ultrasound or computed tomography–guided) may be useful as adjunct measures in addition to antibiotic therapy. (IV—intravenous.)

Medical therapy for tuboovarian abscesses

Clindamycin, 900 mg IV every 8 hrs, *plus*
Gentamicin, 2 mg/kg IV loading dose followed by 1.5 mg/kg
   every 8 hrs
After discharge continue clindamycin, 450 mg orally five times a
   day, to complete a 21-day course
    or
Cefoxitin 2 g IV every 6 hrs, *or*
Cefotetan, 2 g IV every 12 hrs, *plus*
Doxycycline, 100 mg every 12 hrs orally or IV
After discharge continue doxycycline, 100 mg orally
   twice a day to complete a 21-day course

---

*Intravenous therapy should be administered for at least 7 days.

IV—intravenously.

FIGURE 10-20 Medical therapy for tuboovarian abscess. These antibiotic regimens provide adequate coverage against organisms commonly found in tuboovarian abscesses. Specifically, these regimens target anaerobic organisms and both gram-positive and gram-negative aerobic microbes, including *Neisseria gonorrhoeae* and *Chlamydia trachomatis*. The safety of these two regimens is excellent.

Alternative antibiotic regimens for tuboovarian abscesses

Ampicillin/sulbactam, 3 mg IV every 6 hrs, *plus* doxycycline,
   100 mg IV/orally every 12 hrs
Ofloxacin, 400 mg IV twice a day, *plus* either metronidazole,
   500 mg IV every 6 hrs, *or* clindamycin, 900 mg IV every 8 hrs
Imipenem, 500 mg IV every 6 hrs
Ticarcillin/clavulanic acid, 3.1 g IV every 4–6 hrs
Piperacillin/tazobactam, 3.375 g IV every 6 hrs

IV—intravenously.

FIGURE 10-21 Alternative antibiotic regimens for tuboovarian abscesses (TOAs). Given the polymicrobial etiology of TOAs and the importance of anaerobic organisms, broad-spectrum antibiotics achieving adequate tissue levels must be utilized. It must be stressed that there are limited data on these regimens for the treatment of TOAs. There is no current role for outpatient treatment of TOAs, due to concerns of unpredictable gastrointestinal absorption in patients with peritonitis, inadequate tissue levels of antimicrobial agents, and side effects.

A. Response rates of tuboovarian abscesses to medical therapy: Clindamycin plus aminoglycoside

Study	Patients treated, *n*	Patients with response, *n(%)*
Reed *et al.* [3]	64	45 (70)
Landers *et al.* [6]	7	6 (86)
Walker and Gibbs [7]	14	11 (78.6)
Martens *et al.* [8]	16	11 (69)
TOTAL	101	73 (72)

B. Response rates of tuboovarian abscesses to medical therapy: Cefoxitin/cefotetan plus doxycycline

Study	Patients treated, *n*	Patients with response, *n(%)*
Reed *et al.* [3]	37*	31 (84)
Walker and Gibbs [7]	10	9 (90)
Sweet *et al.* [2]	6	4 (67)
Landers *et al.* [6]	9	7 (78)
TOTAL	62	51 (82)

*Five patients received an alternate antibiotic to cefoxitin or cefotetan.

FIGURE 10-22 Response rates of tuboovarian abscesses (TOAs) to medical therapy. **A**, Clindamycin plus aminoglycoside. The combination of clindamycin plus an aminoglycoside is the most commonly used regimen for the treatment of TOAs. Clinical response rate to medical management with broad-spectrum antibiotics is > 70%. **B**, Cefoxitin/cefotetan plus doxycycline.

Second-generation cephalosporins have extended coverage against anaerobic organisms. Cefoxitin or cefotetan-based regimens are appropriate for polymicrobial infections, such as acute pelvic inflammatory disease and TOAs. There is little experience with other second- and third-generation cephalosporins in the treatment of TOAs [2,3,6–8].

Indication for laparotomy in tuboovarian abscesses

Rupture
Failure to respond to conservative management
High suspicion of another diagnosis (*eg*, appendicitis)
Postmenopausal women

FIGURE 10-23 Indications for laparotomy in tuboovarian abscesses. Although most cases respond to conservative medical management, operative intervention plays an extremely important role in the management of tuboovarian abscesses. Surgical intervention, typically laparotomy, is advised in cases that fail to respond to medical management within 48 to 72 hours or in those women with a worsening clinical picture. Postmenopausal women often (44%) will have an associated gynecologic malignancy, such as carcinoma of the fallopian tube, and require surgical intervention. Evidence of response includes symptomatic improvement and objective signs of improvement (*eg*, decreased temperature or leukocyte count), not necessarily a complete cure.

Percutaneous drainage of tuboovarian abscesses

Culdocentesis/colpotomy
Ultrasound-guided
Computed-tomography–guided
Laparoscopy

FIGURE 10-24 Percutaneous drainage of tuboovarian abscesses (TOAs). Culdocentesis and other vaginal drainage procedures have high complication rates (*eg*, peritonitis, sepsis) and often require additional surgery. Thus, they are rarely employed in the management of TOAs. Several case reports and small series have reported excellent success rates for percutaneous drainage of TOAs. These procedures may be of value to prevent aggressive surgical intervention in patients deemed to have failures of medical management. The full role of interventional radiology and laparoscopy in the treatment of TOAs is pending further studies.

Drainage for tuboovarian abscesses not responding to medical therapy

Approach	Patients, *n*	Successful cases, %
Transvaginal ultrasound	30	80–100
Computed tomography–guided (percutaneous)	8	88
Laparoscopy	71	90–95

FIGURE 10-25 Drainage as an alternative to laparotomy for tuboovarian abscesses not responding to medical therapy. Several small nonrandomized studies have demonstrated success of drainage procedures for tuboovarian abscesses. Experience with transabdominal, transvaginal, and laparoscopic drainage is limited, but these procedures may be alternatives to laparotomy in select patients failing broad-spectrum antibiotic therapy. Small collections (< 4 cm) may benefit from aspiration, whereas closed suction drains should be used for larger abscesses. Complications of percutaneous drainage procedures are unusual but include spillage of abscess contents, bacteremia, bleeding, and laceration of intestines [5,9–11].

PELVIC ACTINOMYCOSIS

Pelvic actinomycosis and IUD use

Tuboovarian abscesses due to *Actinomyces israelii* typically seen with prolonged IUD use

Approximately 10% of IUD users are colonized with *A. israelii*

Removal of IUD usually eradicates *A. israelii* colonization

IUD—intrauterine device.

FIGURE 10-26 Pelvic actinomycosis and intrauterine device (IUD) use. *Actinomyces israelii* is a gram-positive anaerobic bacteria with a filamentous branching appearance. It commonly colonizes the gastrointestinal tract, and it does not cause invasive disease unless mucosal barriers are interrupted, as in IUD use. There are no data on the ideal approach to the management of women with incidental findings of *A. israelii* colonization. Currently, many authorities recommend removal of the IUD followed by repeat testing for *A. israelii* by Papanicolaou smear in 2 to 3 months [12,13].

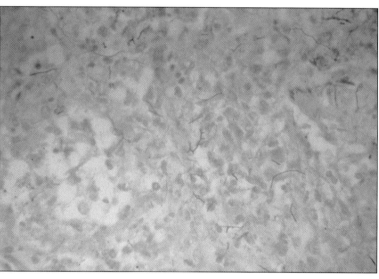

FIGURE 10-27 Histopathologic section demonstrating *Actinomyces israelii* in the wall of a tuboovarian abscess.

Presentation of pelvic actinomycosis

Long latency period

Microabscess formation

Fistula formation

"Woody induration" (characteristic of *Actinomyces israelii*)

Obliteration of tissue planes

FIGURE 10-28 Presentation of pelvic actinomycosis. Pelvic actinomycosis is often not suspected before operative intervention. Its presentation is typically chronic, with the process occurring over several months or years. Abscess formation can be extensive, with obliteration of tissue planes and severe adhesion formation, often mimicking the appearance of gynecologic malignancies.

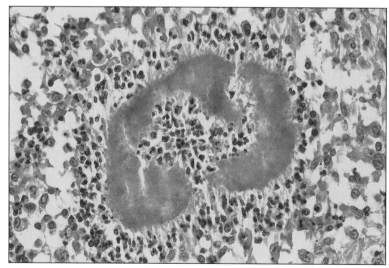

FIGURE 10-29 Sulfur granule in pelvic actinomycosis. The sulfur granule represents colonies of organisms adherent to each other due to a secreted polysaccharide proteinaceous material. Eosinophilic clublike structures extending from the periphery of the sulfur granule can be seen (Splendore-Hoeppli phenomenon).

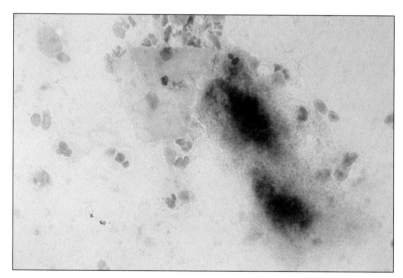

FIGURE 10-30 Papanicolaou smear showing wooly blue-gray masses of *Actinomyces israelii* organisms.

Treatment of pelvic actinomycosis

Removal of the intrauterine device
Surgical excision of the infected tissue
Prolonged course of antibiotics following surgery (6 wks–3 mos)
Penicillin is antibiotic of choice

Figure 10-31 Treatment of pelvic actinomycosis. Excision of infected tissue typically requires total abdominal hysterectomy with bilateral salpino-oophorectomy. Penicillin is the antibiotic of choice given after surgery, but alternatives include the cephalosporins or clindamycin.

REFERENCES

1. Wiesenfeld HC, Sweet RL: Progress in the management of tubo-ovarian abscesses. *Clin Obstet Gynecol* 1993, 36:433–444.

2. Sweet RL, Gibbs RS: Mixed anaerobic-aerobic pelvic infection and pelvic abscess. *In* Sweet SL, Gibbs RS (eds.): *Infectious Diseases of the Female Genital Tract*, 3rd ed. Baltimore: Williams & Wilkins, 1995.

3. Reed SD, Landers DV, Sweet RL: Antibiotic treatment of tubo-ovarian abscess: Comparison of broad spectrum β-lactam agents versus clindamycin-containing regimens. *Am J Obstet Gynecol* 1991, 164:1556–1561.

4. Ginsburg DS, Stern JL, Hamod KA, *et al.*: Tubo-ovarian abscess: A retrospective review. *Am J Obstet Gynecol* 1980, 138(7 pt 2):1055–1058.

5. Henry-Suchet J, Soler A, Loffredo V: Laparoscopic treatment of tuboovarian abscesses. *J Reprod Med* 1984, 29:579–582.

6. Landers DV, Sweet RL: Current trends in the diagnosis and treatment of tubo-ovarian abscesses. *Am J Obstet Gynecol* 1985, 151:1098–1110.

7. Walker CK, Landers DV: Pelvic abscesses: New trends in management. *Obstet Gynecol Surv* 1991, 46:615–624.

8. Martens MG, Faro S, Hammill H: Comparison of cefotaxime, cefoxitin, and clindamycin plus gentamycin in the treatment of uncomplicated and complicated pelvic inflammatory disease. *J Antimicrob Chemother* 1990, 26 (suppl A):37.

9. van Sonnenberg E, D'Agostino HB, Casola G, *et al.*: US-guided transvaginal drainage of pelvic abscesses and fluid collections. *Radiology* 1991, 181:53.

10. Tyrrel RT, Murphy FB, Bernardino ME: Tubo-ovarian abscesses: CT-guided percutaneous drainage. *Radiology* 1990, 175:87.

11. Reich H, McGlynn F: Laparoscopic treatment of tuboovarian and pelvic abscess. *J Reprod Med* 1987, 32:747.

12. Fiorino AS: Intrauterine contraceptive device-associated actinomyces detection on cervical smear. *Obstet Gynecol* 1996, 87:142.

13. Keebler C, Chatwani A, Schwartz R: Actinomycosis infection associated with intrauterine contraceptive devices. *Am J Obstet Gynecol* 1983, 145:596–599.

SELECTED BIBLIOGRAPHY

Keebler C, Chatwani A, Schwartz R: Actinomycosis infection associated with intrauterine contraceptive devices. *Am J Obstet Gynecol* 1983, 145:596–599.

Landers DV, Sweet RL: Current trends in the diagnosis and treatment of tubo-ovarian abscesses. *Am J Obstet Gynecol* 1985, 151:1098–1110.

Reed SD, Landers DV, Sweet RL: Antibiotic treatment of tubo-ovarian abscess: Comparison of broad-spectrum β-lactam agents versus clindamycin-containing regimens. *Am J Obstet Gynecol* 1991, 164:1556–1561.

Sweet RL, Gibbs RS: Mixed anaerobic-aerobic pelvic infection and pelvic abscess. *In* Sweet RL, Gibbs RS (eds.): *Infectious Diseases of the Female Genital Tract*, 3rd ed. Baltimore: Williams & Wilkins; 1995.

Walker CK, Landers DV: Pelvic abscesses: New trends in management. *Obstet Gynecol Surv* 1991, 46:615–624.

Wiesenfeld HC, Sweet RL: Progress in the management of tubo-ovarian abscesses. *Clin Obstet Gynecol* 1993, 36:433–444.

INDEX

A

Abortion
    definition of, 9.2
    mortality in, 9.2
    septic *see* Septic abortion
Abscess
    of kidney, in pyelonephritis, 2.21–2.22
    of ovary *see* Tuboovarian abscess
    perirenal/perinephric
        in diabetes mellitus, 3.10–3.11
        in pyelonephritis, 2.21
    of prostate gland, 4.7–4.8
        treatment of, 4.10–4.11
    tuboovarian *see* Tuboovarian abscess
Actinomyces israelii, in tuboovarian abscess, 10.2, 10.10–10.11
Acyclovir, in cervicitis, 8.19
Adhesions, intrauterine, in septic abortion, 9.7
Adult respiratory distress syndrome, in septic abortion, 9.5
Aerobactin, in pyelonephritis, 2.5
Allergy, vulvar dermatitis in, 7.4
Alpha-blockers, in prostadynia, 4.20
Aminoglycosides, renal pharmacokinetics of, 2.26
Amoxicillin, in pyelonephritis, 2.27
Amoxicillin/clavulanate, in pyelonephritis, 2.27
Amphotericin B
    in cystitis, 5.9–5.10
    in prostatitis, 4.19
    in pyelonephritis, 5.12–5.14
    in urethritis, 5.9–5.10
Ampicillin
    in catheter-associated urinary tract infections, 6.11
    in cystitis, 1.16
    in prostatitis, 4.9
    in pyelonephritis, 2.24–2.26
    in septic abortion, 9.8
Ampicillin/sulbactam, in tuboovarian abscess, 10.8
Angiokeratoma, of vulva, 7.3
Antibiotics
    see also specific antibiotic
    in catheter-associated urinary tract infections, 6.11
        biofilm progress and, 6.8
    in complicated urinary tract infections, 3.3
    in cystitis, 1.15–1.16
    in prostatitis, 4.8–4.10
    in septic abortion, 9.8
Asherman syndrome, in septic abortion, 9.7
Aspergillosis, of urinary tract, 5.15
Autonephrectomy, in tuberculosis, 3.15
Azithromycin
    in cervicitis, 8.19
    in prostatitis, 4.19
Aztreonam
    in pyelonephritis, 2.24, 2.27
    in septic abortion, 9.8

B

Bacteremia, in prostatitis, 4.3, 4.7
Bacterial vaginosis, 7.11, 7.13–7.15
    cervicitis with, 8.9
Bacteriuria
    asymptomatic
        catheter-associated, 6.10
        in diabetes mellitus, 3.9
        in pregnancy, 3.17–3.18
    catheter-associated, 6.5, 6.10
    contraceptive methods and, 1.3
    in elderly persons, 1.4, 1.17
    lifetime frequency of, 1.5
    prevalence of, in elderly persons, 1.4
    sexual intercourse and, 1.3
    in urinary tract infections, diagnostic significance of, 1.6, 1.10
Bartholin's glands, 7.2
Basal cell carcinoma, of vulva, 7.22
Behçet's disease, of vulva, 7.10
Beta-lactam antibiotics, in cystitis, 1.15
Biofilm, in catheter bacterial colonization, 6.7–6.9
Bladder
    calculi of, complicated urinary tract infections in, 3.7
    catheterization of *see* Catheterization;
        Catheter-associated urinary tract infections
    flaccid, complicated urinary tract infections in, 3.8
    host defenses of, against pyelonephritis, 2.4
    infections of *see* Cystitis
    mucosa of, normal, 1.11
    neurogenic, complicated urinary tract infections in, 3.7–3.8
    spastic, complicated urinary tract infections in, 3.8
Blastomycosis
    cystitis in, 5.15
    prostatitis in, 4.17–4.18, 5.15
    pyelonephritis in, 5.15
Bushke-Löwenstein verrucous squamous cell carcinoma, of vulva, 7.20
Butoconazole, in vulvovaginal candidiasis, 7.13

C

Calculi
    complicated urinary tract infections in
        bladder, 3.7
        kidney, 3.4–3.5
        ureter, 3.6
    pyelonephritis in, 2.22
Candida albicans
    in candiduria, 5.2, 5.6
    in pyelonephritis, 3.15
Candida parapsilosis, in candiduria, 5.2
Candida tropicalis, in candiduria, 5.2